Palliative care consultations in primary and metastatic brain tumours

ISTRY LI

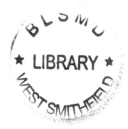

Series information

Series editors

Sara Booth
Macmillan Consultant in Palliative Medicine,
Addenbrooke's Palliative Care Service,
Cambridge, UK

Eduardo Bruera
Professor,
Chair, Department of Palliative Care & Rehabilitation Medicine,
University of Texas M.D. Anderson Cancer Center,
Houston, TX, USA

Advisory editor

Dr. David Oliver
Consultant in Palliative Medicine,
Wisdom Hospice,
Rochester, UK;
and
Honorary Senior Lecturer in Palliative Care,
Kent Institute of Medicine and Health Sciences,
University of Kent, UK

Palliative care consultations in primary and metastatic brain tumours

Sara Booth

Macmillan Consultant in Palliative Medicine,
Addenbrooke's Palliative Care Service,
Cambridge, UK

Eduardo Bruera

Professor,
Chair, Department of Palliative Care & Rehabilitation
Medicine,
University of Texas M.D. Anderson Cancer Center,
Houston, TX, USA

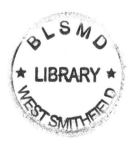

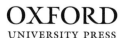

OXFORD
UNIVERSITY PRESS

OXFORD

UNIVERSITY PRESS

Great Clarendon Street, Oxford OX2 6DP

Oxford University Press is a department of the University of Oxford.
It furthers the University's objective of excellence in research, scholarship,
and education by publishing worldwide in

Oxford New York

Auckland Bangkok Buenos Aires Cape Town Chennai
Dar es Salaam Delhi Hong Kong Istanbul Karachi Kolkata
Kuala Lumpur Madrid Melbourne Mexico City Mumbai Nairobi
São Paulo Shanghai Taipei Tokyo Toronto

Oxford is a registered trade mark of Oxford University Press
in the UK and in certain other countries

Published in the United States
by Oxford University Press Inc., New York

© Oxford University Press 2004

The moral rights of the author have been asserted

Database right Oxford University Press (maker)

First published 2004

A catalogue record for this title is available from the British Library

ISBN 0 19 852807 8 (Pbk)

10 9 8 7 6 5 4 3 2 1

Typeset by Newgen Imaging Systems (P) Ltd., Chennai, India
Printed in Great Britain
on acid-free paper by
Biddles Ltd, King's Lynn

Palliative Care Consultations Series Foreword

Professor M A Richards
National Cancer Director, England

Despite the significant advances in diagnosis and treatment that have been made in recent decades, cancer remains a major cause of death in all developed countries. It is therefore essential that all health professionals who provide direct care for cancer patients should be aware of what can be done to alleviate suffering.

Major progress has been made over the past thirty years or so in the relief of physical symptoms and in approaches to the delivery of psychological, social, and spiritual care for cancer patients and their families and carers. However, the problems of providing holistic care should not be underestimated. This is particularly the case in busy acute general hospitals and cancer centres. The physical environment may not be conducive to the care of a dying patient. Staff may have difficulty recognizing the point at which radical interventions are no longer in a patient's best interests, when the emphasis should change to care with palliative intent.

Progress in the treatment of cancer has also led to many patients who, although incurable, live for years with their illness. They may have repeated courses of treatment and some will have a significant burden of symptoms that must be optimally controlled.

One of the most important developments in recent years has been the recognition of the benefits of a multidisciplinary or multiprofessional approach to cancer care. Physicians, surgeons, radiologists, haematologists, pathologists, oncologists, palliative care specialists, nurse specialists, and a wide range of other health professionals all have major contributions to make. These specialists need to work together in teams.

One of the prerequisites for effective teamwork is that individual members should recognize the contribution that others can make. The *Palliative Care Consultations* series should help to make this a reality. The editors are to be congratulated in bringing together distinguished cancer and palliative care specialists from all parts of the world. Individual volumes focus predominantly on the problems faced by patients with a particular type of cancer (e.g. breast or lung) or groups of cancers (e.g. haematological malignancies or gynaecological cancers). The chapters of each volume set out what can be achieved using anti-cancer treatments and through the delivery of palliative care.

I warmly welcome the series and I believe the individual volumes will prove valuable to a wide range of clinicians involved in the delivery of high quality care.

Contents

Contributors

Mohammad Z. Al-Shahri
Consultant, Palliative Medicine,
Department of Oncology,
King Faisal Specialist Hospital and
Research Center,
Riyadh,
Saudi Arabia

Terri S. Armstrong
Department of Neuro-Oncology,
University of Texas MD Anderson
Cancer Center,
Houston, Texas,
USA

V. Ramesh Bulusu
Neuro-Oncology Unit,
Oncology Centre,
Addenbrooke's Hospital,
Cambridge,
UK

Neil G. Burnet
Neuro-Oncology Unit,
University of Cambridge,
Department of Oncology and
Oncology Centre,
Addenbrooke's Hospital,
Cambridge,
UK

P. Edmonds
Consultant in Palliative Medicine,
King's College Hospital NHS Trust,
London,
UK

Robin L. Fainsinger
Associate Professor,
Division of Palliative Medicine,
Department of Oncology,
University of Alberta,
Edmonton, Alberta,
Canada

E. J. Hall
Specialist Registrar in Palliative
Medicine,
London (South) and KSS Training
Scheme,
UK

Sarah J. Jefferies
Neuro-Oncology Unit,
Oncology Centre,
Addenbrooke's Hospital,
Cambridge,
UK

Anne E. Kayl
Department of Neuro-Oncology,
The University of Texas MD
Anderson Cancer Center,
Houston, Texas,
USA

Annette Landy
Head of Psychological Support
Services,
Specialist Palliative Care Unit,
Arthur Rank House,
Cambridge,
UK

Linda Launchbury
Macmillan Clinical Nurse Specialist
(Palliative Care),
Peterborough District Hospital,
UK

F. A. Malik
Specialist Registrar in Palliative
Medicine,
London (South) and KSS Training
Scheme,
UK

Christina A. Meyers
Department of Neuro-Oncology,
The University of Texas MD
Anderson Cancer Center,
Houston, Texas,
USA

David Oliver
Consultant in Palliative Medicine,
Wisdom Hospice, High Bank,
Rochester, Kent,
UK
and
Honorary Senior Lecturer in
Palliative Care,
Kent Institute of Medicine and
Health Sciences, University of Kent,
UK

Vinay K. Puduvalli
Department of Neuro-Oncology,
University of Texas MD
Anderson Cancer Center,
Houston, Texas,
USA

Odette Spruyt
Director of Pain and Palliative
Care Services,
Peter MacCallum Cancer Institute,
Melbourne,
Australia

Helen White
Specialist Speech and Language
Therapist,
Royal Marsden Hospital, Sutton,
UK

Chapter 1

Management of primary brain tumours

Neil G. Burnet, V. Ramesh Bulusu, and Sarah J. Jefferies

Introduction

Neuro-oncology is a particularly difficult area, for patients, family, and staff alike. The gliomas are amongst the most devastating of all cancers, and our patients face some unique problems. From the point of view of workload, including palliative and supportive care, the work appears dominated by high-grade gliomas. Indeed, palliative and supportive care play an essential role in the management of almost all patients with high-grade gliomas at some time in the illness, so that the overlap between neuro-oncology and palliative care is larger than most areas of oncology (see Fig. 1.1).

Primary CNS tumours affect patients of all ages, from childhood to old age, with a bimodal distribution of incidence with age, with a peak in early childhood, a trough in the teens to mid-twenties, and then a steady rise with older age. They are the most prevalent solid tumours of childhood, and indeed the second leading cancer-related cause of death in children. They are the third leading cancer-related cause of death in adolescents and adults between 15 and 35. Primary CNS tumours account for about 2% of all primary tumours. In absolute numbers, therefore, these tumours represent a minor problem in oncology. However, CNS tumours actually cause the greatest loss of life of any of the adult tumours. This can be computed as the 'average years of life lost': brain tumours account for an average of 20 years of life lost per affected patient, greater than all of the common solid tumours, including, for example, lung, breast, or prostate cancer. In this sense, brain tumours represent a very significant problem in hospital, hospice, primary care, and society.

Our unit sees approximately 200 new patients with primary CNS tumours each year. The majority are gliomas, which represents two-thirds of our work (see Fig. 1.2). High-grade gliomas, that is grade III and grade IV tumours together, constitute just over half of our referrals, but grade IV glioma,

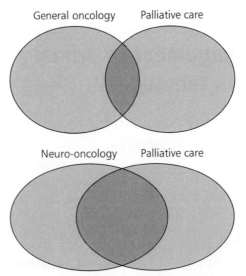

Fig. 1.1 The relationship between oncology and palliative medicine, showing the greater overlap with neuro-oncology.

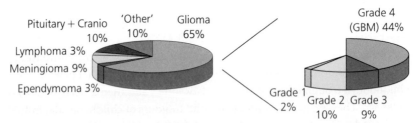

Fig. 1.2 The distribution of diagnoses in our practice: 10% of cases are shown as 'Other'. These represent the surprisingly numerous rare types of primary tumour, which individually are few in number, and a few patients with metastases in whom the primary tumour cannot be found. In the category 'Pituitary + Cranio', pituitary adenomas constitute for 8% and craniopharyngiomas account for the additional 2%.

i.e. glioblastoma multiforme (GBM), is by far the most common: we see five grade IV gliomas for every grade III.

These devastating tumours consume much of our energy and indeed resources, and have a major emotional impact on staff. It is important to remember that one third of our neuro-oncology cases have alternative diagnoses, so that resources must be balanced appropriately. It is also important to note that some primary CNS tumours are eminently curable, and these patients need to be treated carefully and encouraged to look forward to the future. Germinoma, for example, is rare in adults but should have a cure rate of almost 100%. These tumours sometimes produce very rapid neurological deterioration, so that radiotherapy may need to be started as an emergency, since steroids alone may not be sufficient. Medulloblastoma should be curable in about 60% of patients, perhaps in a greater proportion with the introduction of adjuvant chemotherapy. In both of these conditions, obsessional attention to details of radiotherapy is vital in ensuring successful outcome. Ependymoma is curable in about 50% of patients.

In patients with tumours other than gliomas, indications for radiotherapy are still increasing. For example, the role of radiotherapy in the management of meningioma is now more widely appreciated, so that more patients are being referred. Radiotherapy also plays a role in the management of patients with acoustic schwannoma (often known as acoustic neuroma). Some patients are treated with stereotactic radiosurgery but others are more appropriately treated with fractionated (stereotactic conformal) radiotherapy. Ten percent of our referrals are for patients with pituitary lesions, either pituitary adenoma (8%) or craniopharyngioma (2%). These patients require life-long endocrine follow-up but do not usually require palliative services.

Figure 1.2 shows that 10% of cases have a diagnosis of 'other', and these cases represent the surprisingly numerous but rare types of primary tumour, which individually are few in number. Only a few patients with metastases are included here. The majority of patients with metastases in our centre are referred directly to the appropriate site-specific teams, and only the small minority whose primary tumour cannot be found are managed by the neuro-oncology team. This chapter does not address the management of patients with brain metastases, nor children with primary brain tumours.

The roles of the neuro-oncologist include:

- patient care—active treatment and palliation;
- treatment development—improving tumour control and reducing side-effects;
- research—we do not want to have the same dismal outcomes in another 5 years.

Particularly in the context of high-grade gliomas, where the outlook is so poor, treatment development and research are essential if we are to make progress. There has been some improvement in side-effect profiles over the last 20 years but no real progress in tumour control. It would be a tragedy if we have not improved both areas in the next 20 years.

Problems unique to patients with brain tumours

A number of problems exist in patients with brain tumours that are unique or nearly so. The first major problem is one of intellectual and personality change. This is quite different even from advanced systemic tumours, unless cerebral metastases supervene. This can be one of the most distressing consequences of the condition. Motor disorders occur and particular difficulty is hemiplegia, which again is rare in other tumours without CNS metastases. Seizures occur, although in most cases these are controllable with modern medication. The side-effects of medications, especially dexamethasone, are also unique (see below). Dexamethasone is associated with muscle wasting, which in association with weight gain is particularly problematic. There is a surprising variation in the severity of side-effects between different patients taking the same dexamethasone dose. For some, quite low doses produce tremendous weight gain and muscle wasting; for others, moderate doses are tolerated without these problems, sometimes for a surprisingly long time.

Types of primary CNS tumours

Primary brain tumours can broadly be divided into primary glial tumours, medulloblastoma, ependymoma, germ cell tumours (germinoma and teratoma), meningioma, nerve sheath tumours (such as acoustic schwannoma), and pituitary tumours—see Table 1.1. Most of these tumours can also affect the spinal cord.

The glial tumours are graded from I to IV; grades I and II together constitute low-grade glioma (LGG), while grades III and IV comprise high-grade glioma (HGG). Grade I tumours typically occur in childhood and are rare in adults. They are on occasion more malignant than their low-grade designation would suggest and cannot necessarily be regarded as benign. Grade II tumours, that is astrocytoma, oligodendroglioma, and mixed oligo-astrocytomas, have a much better outlook than their high-grade counterparts. A grade III designation of these tumours leads to the term 'anaplastic' to precede the specific name, such as anaplastic astrocytoma. A grade IV glial tumour is a glioblastoma multiforme (GBM), regardless of the cell of origin.

Treatment of non-glial tumours

As noted above, there are conditions requiring radiotherapy over and above the glial tumours, and the indications for radiotherapy are still increasing. For example, more patients with meningioma are now referred for radiotherapy in order to prevent recurrence. Classification of these tumours has become more specific and this aids the decision concerning post-operative radiotherapy.

Table 1.1 Major categories of primary brain tumours

Glial tumours
Astrocytoma Oligodendroglioma Oligo-astrocytoma
Medulloblastoma
Ependymoma
Germinoma/teratoma
Meningioma
Nerve sheath tumours (e.g. acoustic schwannoma)
Pituitary adenoma and craniopharyngioma

Notes:
1. The glial tumours are divided in to four grades: grade I and II together constitute low-grade gliomas (LGGs) while grade III and IV tumours together are the high grade gliomas (HGGs). Grade I tumours are rare in adults, though they do occur. They also appear in adult practice in patients treated as children who have outgrown the paediatric services.
2. Considering the HGGs, the term 'anaplastic' attached to a specific tumour type is the same as specifying a grade III tumour of that type. The term glioblastoma multiforme (GBM) is the synonym for grade IV tumours, from whatever cell type they originally arose. Gliosarcomas are a subset of GBM, though it is not clear whether their behaviour differs or not.

Radiotherapy is increasingly used for the treatment of acoustic schwannomas, where it is extremely effective. Pituitary adenomas represent an important use of radiotherapy as an adjunct to surgery, and craniopharyngioma, which occurs in the same region, should be referred for radiotherapy as well. In all of these conditions, modern developments in radiotherapy, such as conformal and stereotactic radiotherapy, have led to an improvement in outcome, particularly by improving normal tissue side-effects.

The gliomas

The rest of this chapter will be devoted to the major problem of patients with malignant gliomas. In this context, the term 'radical' means 'with curative intent', while 'palliative' describes treatment designed to alleviate symptoms, though with no prospect of cure.

Low-grade gliomas

The initial management of patients with grade II gliomas can be difficult, specifically in knowing whether or not to investigate with a biopsy or surgical resection. Once the diagnosis of glioma has been confirmed with histology, there is a second decision to be made regarding further treatment. In oncology centres, most patients are considered for further treatment because they are usually referred when symptoms or signs are worsening. As well as neurological deterioration, worsening seizure control or imaging may indicate progressive tumour. In these circumstances further treatment is to be recommended. Radiotherapy appears the most effective and sustained treatment, and therefore it is our practice to recommend radiotherapy as the first treatment after an appropriate surgical procedure. Results in our department show that the 1-year survival for patients with grade II gliomas treated radically is around 98%, 2-year survival is 87%, and 3- and 5-year survival is 79% (see Fig. 1.3). The introduction of conformal radiotherapy, which spares substantial amounts of normal brain, has reduced the acute and late complications of radiotherapy and make it a well-tolerated treatment, in the short and long term.

There is now good evidence from a European randomized controlled trial that the timing of radiotherapy does not affect the overall survival. This study randomized patients to receive radiotherapy at the time of presentation or for this to be deferred until progression of tumour. Overall survival was the same in both arms. However, the disease-free survival, that is the period of optimum neurological performance, was longer in those patients assigned to the

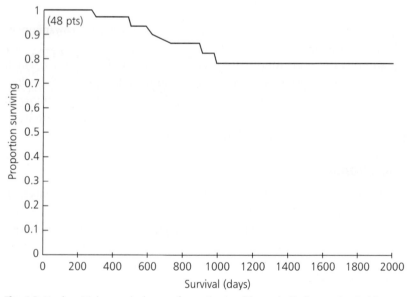

Fig. 1.3 Kaplan–Meier survival curve for patients with grade II gliomas treated in our unit. Complete data are currently available for 48 cases.

early radiotherapy arm. This is the major reason that we recommend early radiotherapy to patients, where this choice is available. Chemotherapy has been used to good effect in patients with low-grade tumours. However, responses occur in only about 60% of patients, and although some of these responses are quite long, most patients will subsequently progress. If this is given as initial treatment, most patients have to go on to have radiotherapy later.

Grade II tumours typically grow by infiltration into normal functioning brain. This means that complete surgical resection is usually inappropriate and impossible. Typically these tumours infiltrate but do not expand like an inflated balloon. There is usually no central mass of tumour, which expands and destroys the surrounding brain. This pattern of growth is important for planning treatment. It also explains why these tumours can become quite substantial in size but often cause surprisingly mild neurological deficit. Radiotherapy often improves symptoms and signs, and sometimes this occurs even during the course of the treatment. It is very important to recognize that this is a common situation: even in circumstances where the outlook for the patient appears poor, radiotherapy may still be appropriate to try to improve disabling neurology.

Radiotherapy may also improve seizures in patients with low-grade tumours and may be a useful adjunct to anticonvulsants. One large study found improvement in about two-thirds of patients. In some cases, this is a major reason for proceeding to radiotherapy. Imaging after radiotherapy usually demonstrates surprisingly little change, though over a period of months to years there may be slight reduction in size. The reason for this is the growth pattern of diffuse infiltration. This can be confusing to patients and it is useful for the patient to be aware that imaging will not only not return to normal, but may hardly change. Following treatment, grade II tumours may relapse. These relapses may occur with the same growth characteristics as the original tumour, but about 50% transform to a higher grade, grade III or more often grade IV, when their behaviour and outcome becomes much more aggressive. It is often suggested that radiotherapy induces such transformation but there is good evidence against this.

Low-grade glioma: case histories

Case 1 A right-handed young man of 22 presented with seizures, some associated word-finding difficulty, and some incoordination of the right side, due to a left temporo-parietal tumour. Biopsy confirmed the diagnosis of grade II oligodendroglioma. He was treated with radical radiotherapy, which improved his neurological function, and reduced the severity and frequency of his seizures. He remains well 6 years after treatment.

Case 2 By contrast, a young woman of 26 with a grade II astrocytoma presented with headache, confusion, and deteriorating vision. This lesion occupied much of one hemisphere of the brain, impairing her vision through involvement of the optic radiation. Her symptoms were progressing rapidly, and the headache in particular proved difficult to control. Radiotherapy was therefore started urgently, to treat most of the cerebrum. Her headaches began to improve shortly after the commencement of radiotherapy, and the visual deterioration was arrested and subsequently improved. Confusion also improved during the radiotherapy treatment. Following completion of treatment she remained well and was able to return to work. About 1 year after completion of treatment she unfortunately relapsed. She was then treated with palliative chemotherapy with useful response for a further year before the tumour progressed again. At this point her vision failed and she developed hemiplegia, so that her final illness was complicated by these difficult deficits before she finally succumbed to her illness.

Analysis

These cases represent the extremes of outcome for patients with LGG. The long survival of most patients with these tumours (Fig. 1.3) is a major consideration in the use of modern radiotherapy technologies, which minimize both acute and late side-effects. Reduction in seizures was an important benefit for the first case.

In the second case, radiotherapy was effective in improving the neurological deficits. This is common in patients with LGG, but rare in patients with HGG. In order to maximize this benefit, as well as for the benefit of symptom control, radiotherapy was started urgently. Tumour progression occurred later, probably without transformation to a higher histological grade. This demonstrates that the current histological classification is not a complete description of behaviour. Useful palliation was achieved with chemotherapy. However, the final phase of her illness required extensive palliative care, because of blindness and hemiplegia.

High-grade gliomas

These represent just over half of the neuro-oncology referrals (Fig. 1.2). There is a substantial difference in outcome between grade III and grade IV tumours. For grade III tumours, the median survival is around 3 years in our unit; whilst for grade IV tumours, the median survival is just over 9 months—see Table 1.2. We see five patients with glioblastoma multiforme (GBM) for every one with a grade III tumour. As is usual for malignancy, there is a male predominance of 1.4 : 1. The prognostic factors for outcome are shown in Table 1.3.

Table 1.2 Survival data for just over 300 adult patients with high-grade glioma treated in our unit from 1996 to 2001

Treatment intent	Survival			
	Median (days)	1 year (%)	2 year (%)	3 year (%)
Radical				
Grade III	1150	73	57	53
Grade IV	279	38	8	3
Palliative	140	12	7	0
Supportive	43	3	1	0

Notes:

1. The prognosis of each treatment group is critically dependent on the selection criteria. More stringent criteria for both radical and palliative treatments actually improves the outcome in all categories—a case of the 'Will Rogers' phenomenon.

2. The overall median survival of high grade glioma patients treated radically, considering grade III and IV cases together, is 315 days. This reflects the preponderance of grade IV tumours, with an approximate 5:1 ratio.

3. Median survival is the best single parameter to describe population survival; unlike the mean, it avoids being biased by a small number of long term survivors. Typically, mean survival is longer than median for this reason. For the long survivors, in the 'tail' of the population survival curve, the 2 year or 3-year survival rate is more useful.

4. In this context, the term 'radical' means 'with curative intent', while 'palliative' describes treatment designed to means to alleviate symptoms but with no prospect of cure.

Table 1.3 Prognostic factors for adult patients with high-grade glioma treated radically

Age
WHO performance status
Extent of surgery
Length of history of fits (the longer the better)
Grade—grade III versus grade IV
Location of the tumour
Tumour growth rate—not measurable
Tumour response to radiotherapy and chemotherapy—not measurable

Notes:

1. The Medical Research Council (MRC) studied prognostic factors, and developed a prognostic index. Their studies did not find grade a significant prognostic factor, probably due to difficulties in classification. The newer WHO 2000 pathology classification is more reproducible, and shows a large difference depending on grade—see Fig. 1.4, p. 20.

2. Extent of surgery is important. Surgical resection is valuable both to improve survival, but it also facilitates radiotherapy—dexamethasone doses can be lower, and side-effects are significantly less.

One of the most difficult issues in dealing with brain tumours is the initial decision about how to manage the patient. When the patient is first seen, a decision must be made to recommend radical treatment, palliative treatment, or supportive care alone. Typical schedules are shown in Table 1.4. In general, this decision is based on two main factors: age and performance status (see Table 1.5). In terms of age, different units have different cut-off ages for accepting patients for radical treatment. In our unit, patients of 70 and above are not offered radical radiotherapy. This is not designed to be an age-ist strategy but rather to improve the care of older patients in a specific and deliberate way. The general effects of radical radiotherapy in elderly patients are much more severe, and experience shows that HGG patients over 70 treated with radical radiotherapy experience much worse acute side-effects than younger patients. This treatment strategy therefore represents a poor 'buy' for such patients. There is also a suggestion that high-grade tumours in elderly patients may grow more rapidly on average than those in younger patients, so that rapid access to treatment, which is usually possible for palliative radiotherapy (but often not for radical treatment), may be an added advantage. Performance status is the other major criterion for accepting patients for radical radiotherapy. In general, we only accept patients in whom there is no significant neurological abnormality. This appears to be a very clear cut criterion, in theory, but in practice it may be harder to apply than it first appears—'The difference between theory and practice is bigger in practice than in theory'.

Table 1.4 Typical radiotherapy schedules for patients with glioma

Radical
- 54–60 Gy
- 30 fractions
- 6 weeks, treating 5 days per week, Monday to Friday
- CT planning, with or without MRI as needed

Palliative
- 30 Gy
- 6 fractions
- 2 weeks, treating 3 days per week, typically Monday, Wednesday & Friday
- Simulator planning

Notes:
1. The SI unit of radiotherapy dose is the gray (after the physicist Dr L. H. Gray), abbreviated to Gy. The effects of a course of radiotherapy depend on the total dose, but also the dose per fraction and the overall treatment time.

Table 1.5 Selection criteria for different treatment strategies

Radical

- Fit—performance Status (PS) 0, or occasionally 1
- Age <70

Palliative

- Less fit—PS 2, and age <70
- Fit—PS 0 or 1, and age 70 or more

Supportive care

- Major neurological defect

Notes:
1. Patient and family preference, and social context are also critical in decision-making for treatment options.
2. Acceptance criteria for each category actually alter outcome. If the acceptance criteria for treatment are more stringent, more of the better prognosis patients fall into each of the three categories, leading to an improvement in outcome in *all* categories. This is known colloquially as the 'Will Rogers' phenomenon.

Obvious deficits that should preclude radical radiotherapy are confusion or hemiplegia. However, how should these criteria be applied to a patient with a homonomous hemianopia due to a posterior parietal non-dominant hemisphere lesion? The reason that such a patient has neurological disturbance is purely related to the location of the tumour. In this case, we would probably accept the patient for radical radiotherapy, in part because movement deficits or confusion may be associated with worse outcome. It may also be difficult to know how to advise a patient with an expressive dysphasia. Such patients may have normal intellect and can communicate by answering questions, though they may not be able to form words or sentences themselves. This clearly represents a significant neurological deficit but these patients survive better than those with, for example, hemiplegia. In our unit, patients are accepted for palliative treatment if they have modest deficit or if they are fit but 70 or over. We recommend supportive care for patients with severe deficit, for whom there is a 'lose–lose' situation. Since these tumours typically cause irreversible neurological damage, successful treatment may not improve neurology and hence not improve the quality of life (see also below). In a patient with a severe neurological deficit, successful palliative radiotherapy treatment, with shrinkage of the tumour and subsequent growth delay, may simply leave the patient with a poor quality of life for longer. Unsuccessful treatment, that is with the radiotherapy affecting the tumour to a minimal extent, subjects the patient to unnecessary treatment, only a modest intrusion into quality of life, but without any subsequent gain. This may be a useful way of explaining the disadvantage of treatment to the patient themselves and to their family. The patient and family need to be involved in the decision-making on treatment options. This may need considerable time, from medical and nursing staff. Our policy is to try to explain the merits of the appropriate treatment choice, and to avoid disagreements or confrontation. In the long run, it is always better for the patient and family to believe that the medical team is working with, not against, them. Occasionally, there is real uncertainty about the treatment options for the patient and family, particularly in choosing between palliative radiotherapy or supportive care alone. In this situation a 2-week interval before another appointment can be very helpful. It gives time for them to review the options and shows whether or not the patient is deteriorating already, a strong indication to avoid radiotherapy.

In our unit, about half of the patients with high-grade glioma are taken on for radical radiotherapy; about a third receive palliative radiotherapy, leaving about one-sixth to receive supportive care alone. In *all* cases appropriate support should be offered; this is appreciated by patients and their carers. Amongst those patients treated radically, a few patients appear to be cured. In our experience this proportion is about 1%, though the survival rate at 3 years is 3%. Unfortunately, this indicates that two out of three patients who survive for 3 years will eventually succumb from tumour. Nevertheless, these survivors are important, especially in relation to potential long-term side-effects.

The acceptance criteria for radical radiotherapy vs. palliative, or palliate vs. supportive care, may have a profound effect on the outcome of the whole patient group. By making acceptance criteria in the two treatment categories more stringent, more of the better prognosis patients fall into each of the three categories. This actually improves the average outcome in *all* categories. This is analogous to the phenomenon of improved staging methods leading to improved outcome and is known colloquially as the 'Will Rogers' phenomenon.

Growth pattern and growth rate of high-grade gliomas

HGGs typically grow with two different components. The central part of the tumour expands like an inflating balloon, destroying surrounding brain and leading to irreversible neurological damage. This is usually delineated by contrast-enhancing abnormality on CT or MRI. Around this area is a front of microscopic infiltration, which can be very extensive. Typically, this infiltration occurs without necessarily causing irreversible damage, though it does produce significant oedema. The extent of the oedema probably exceeds the extent of tumour cell infiltration. Treatment with steroids will often reverse the symptoms or neurological deficit caused by the oedema, and gives a good idea of the ultimate maximum neurological function that the patient can expect. This microscopic infiltration is the reason that radical surgery is not curative. It also needs to be taken into account when treating patients with radiotherapy. Delays to start radiotherapy present a significant problem, including stress on neuro-oncology staff. It has been demonstrated that, on average, a 4-week delay in starting radiotherapy leads to a 10-week reduction in median survival.[1] Our own work on the growth rate of HGGs suggests that, from the time of presentation, a quarter of tumours double in volume in 30 days or less. Since this volume increase comes after presentation, when neurological symptoms and signs have already developed, it can be very significant. Thus, delays to start treatment may be a major disadvantage to a proportion of patients. This further confuses the choice between radical radiotherapy, which often takes 6 or more weeks to begin, and palliative radiotherapy, which usually starts in our unit within 5–14 days.

The delay to start radical radiotherapy, which is the result of chronic national under-resourcing of oncology services, has led us to start using chemotherapy while waiting to start radiotherapy. This 'neoadjuvant' application of chemotherapy should confer a benefit for some patients, with minimal toxicity. Despite this, occasional patients taken on for radical radiotherapy deteriorate while waiting for radiotherapy. If this happens, it is better to proceed to immediate palliative radiotherapy rather than continue with the delay. It is important to explain the problem to the patient and family, but most understand the value of the change having seen neurology worsen. The relatively high palliative dose given in 2 weeks rather than 6 (Table 1.4) is a genuine advantage in treating rapidly progressive tumours.

Chemotherapy for glioma

The first- and second-line chemotherapy schedules for patients with glioma are shown in Table 1.6. In general, these are tolerated reasonably well. Responses are seen in about one third of patients, though lower grade tumours respond better, and responses to second line treatment may be worse. For neoadjuvant chemotherapy we use the first line PCV schedule.

An interesting and distressing problem associated with the need to formally assess chemotherapy response is that a proportion of patients are found on routine imaging to have progression, without necessarily having experienced significant neurological deficit. Where this happens on first-line chemotherapy, a switch can be made to second-line treatment. When further progression is found on imaging, the situation is especially distressing because no effective third-line treatment is available.

Table 1.6 Standard chemotherapy schedules, as per the NICE guidelines

First-line—three agents PCV chemotherapy
• Procarbazine orally, daily for 10 days
• CCNU orally, as a single dose
• Vincristine intravenously, as a short out-patient infusion
• Repeat 6 weekly
Second-line—single agent temozolomide (trade name Temodal)
• Temozolomide orally, daily for 5 days
• Repeat 4 weekly

Notes:
1. Switch to second-line chemotherapy in the face of either progression of tumour or unacceptable side-effects.
2. Review clinical progress and imaging (CT or MR) after every three courses.
3. Treatment is usually given for 9–12 months provided tumour response is maintained and side-effects are acceptable. Occasionally treatment may go on for longer.
4. There is currently no third-line chemotherapy that is particularly effective.

High-grade glioma: case histories

Case 1 A right-handed 38-year-old mother of three presented with right-sided weakness, and expressive dysphasia. A large tumour was seen in the left frontal region, involving the motor cortex. Initially, biopsy had been performed to prove the diagnosis of GBM. Her symptoms and signs improved on dexamethasone but then worsened rapidly, so radiotherapy was commenced urgently. However, this led to raised intra-cranial pressure, with headache, confusion, worsening of the dysphasia, and right-sided weakness. Urgent craniotomy was therefore carried out, with considerable improvement in all symptoms and signs. Radiotherapy was restarted 3 days after surgery, and completed as planned, by which time she had good comprehension of speech with only a mild expressive dysphasia, but marked right-sided weakness, amounting to functional hemiplegia. Over the next 12 months her neurological deficits improved slightly, and she herself was pleased to be involved with her family. A further 12 months on she developed progressive neurology, with complete hemiplegia and aphasia. Palliative chemotherapy, initiated at the request of the patient and her husband, stabilized her condition for around 6 months (30 months after presentation), when she began to decline again. She survived for a further 6 months requiring nursing care, initially at home then in her local hospice before dying 3 years after presentation.

Case 2 A man of 53 presented with headaches, which lead to imaging, followed by craniotomy and debulking of a frontal lobe GBM. He had no neurological deficit following surgery. Radical radiotherapy was started as soon as possible, and was well tolerated until the last week of treatment, when he became exhausted, weak, and lethargic. Although no hard neurological signs were present, he had clearly deteriorated significantly in terms of activities of daily living. CT scanning was not helpful in distinguishing acute radiotherapy effects from early recurrence. However, his neurological function continued to deteriorate, he became bed-bound 1 month after completing radiotherapy, and died 5 months later from progressive tumour.

Case 3 A woman of 32, with two young children, presented with a short history of headache and right-sided weakness, which were progressive. Imaging revealed a tumour suspicious of a grade IV glioma (GBM). Craniotomy and debulking was performed, and histology confirmed the diagnosis. Postoperatively her deficit resolved. Because of the relatively rapid progression of her neurology pre-operatively, her radiotherapy was planned urgently using a simple though crude technique, and treatment commenced within 14 days of her first oncology consultation, and 19 days after her craniotomy. After 2 weeks her treatment was changed to a CT-based radiotherapy plan, and she received a standard radical radiotherapy dose (Table 1.4). Just over 5 years later she remains well, working full-time and with no sign of recurrence. Her hair has regrown almost normally. She attends for follow-up once a year, with some anxiety, for simple endocrine assessment of her hypothalamic-pituitary axis.

Analysis

Case 1 appears to show different selection criteria for radical radiotherapy. However, this case was muddied by the rapid deterioration, from an initially excellent performance status. The patient was also insistent on her wish to maximize survival. Paradoxically, the rapid deterioration allowed urgent commencement of treatment so that the normal disadvantage of delay for radical radiotherapy did not occur. This case also illustrates the value of debulking surgery, to decompress threatened areas of the brain and permit radiotherapy to be completed. Chemotherapy delivered useful palliation and prolongation of life for her, though intensive palliative care support was required. Treatment in this case allowed her an additional 3 years of life with her family, with what she judged to be acceptable quality of life.

Case 2 illustrates some of the difficulties of early recurrence after radiotherapy. For the patient, the investment of 6 weeks of treatment time may seem to have been wasted. It also illustrates the problem of accurate diagnosis of early recurrence, which can be problematic. Despite early recurrence, death was surprisingly delayed. Cases that show this resistance to treatment are psychologically devastating for all concerned, but fortunately are uncommon.

Case 3 is included to show that some patients do survive in the long term; she has probably been cured. Careful attention to radiotherapy details is worthwhile to maximize the effectiveness of treatment and minimize the toxicity. This includes commencing treatment as fast as possible (see section on 'Growth pattern and growth rate of high-grade gliomas'), and using sophisticated planning techniques. Long-term follow-up is also necessary.

Presentation of patients with primary brain tumours

Initial presentation

Patients with primary brain tumours typically present with one or more of the following symptom types:

- headache
- seizures
- neurological deficit
- tiredness.

The majority of primary brain tumours in adults occur in the supratentorial region and are associated with relatively localized abnormalities. In some patients, headache can be quite severe, though it is rarely a problem later in the course of the illness.

A few patients also present with a general fatigue. Although shown in the list above, this is not a well-described feature of brain tumours. Clearly, a patient attending his or her GP complaining of tiredness is not likely to arouse the suspicion of a glioma. Nevertheless, this is the presenting complaint in a number of patients, and in many more, tiredness develops through the course of the illness and can be a significant symptom with important negative effects on quality of life. Much less common, is a set of symptoms associated with acute obstructive hydrocephalus, which is usually secondary to tumours in the posterior fossa, less commonly in the region of the pineal gland, which obstruct the aqueduct. In this case, headache can be severe and is often associated with projectile vomiting. There may also be drowsiness, confusion, and ataxia. This is a specific problem related to mass effect causing CSF flow obstruction. Very occasionally tumours in the frontal lobe obstruct the foramen of Monro (connecting the lateral ventricles to the third ventricle), causing hydrocephalus in one or both lateral ventricles. This produces a less severe clinical picture. CSF obstruction is usually managed surgically, either by insertion of a ventriculo-peritoneal (VP) shunt or occasionally by a third ventriculostomy.

Presentation at relapse

A useful rule of thumb is that gliomas typically recapitulate the symptoms of the initial presentation when they relapse. It is obvious that a patient noticing worsening neurological function is likely to have progressive tumour. Patients will usually describe alteration of their ability to carry out the activities of daily living. This is usually a more sensitive indicator of potential problems than a rapid clinical examination, particularly where hard neurological signs have been present for some time. Seizures may also worsen, with increasing frequency and severity. It is useful to remember that symptoms of recurrence normally mirror initial symptoms, even if these are not entirely typical and the pathophysiology not understood. For example, small, localized recurrences without major mass effect can still produce headache. Why this should occur is not clear but it is an important phenomenon, which needs to be taken seriously. Although headache may be associated with recurrence, it is usually localized and mild. For reasons that are not clear, headache is rarely a problem later, in patients with recurrent glioma. It is relatively uncommon even to need analgesia over and above simple non-steroidal drugs. However, in rare cases where headache is severe, it can normally be managed using standard opioid analgesics. Dexamethasone is a useful adjunct in the management of the symptoms of recurrence. It may even help seizures, although it does not have specific anticonvulsant properties. Its mode of action is presumably mediated through reduction of oedema surrounding the tumour or membrane stabilization.

Symptoms not caused by relapse

However, there are *other* causes of symptoms that suggest recurrence. Seizures may worsen if anticonvulsant control has been lost. This is rarely the result of non-compliance; it is more commonly due to confusion about doses. Tiredness, lethargy, mild confusion, and ataxia may indicate phenytoin toxicity. The conclusion is that anticonvulsants should be carefully monitored.

Early deterioration after radical radiotherapy

A number of patients experience early deterioration after the completion of treatment. This can be a surprisingly difficult problem to elucidate, and can be related either to side-effects of treatment, which will settle with time, or to early progression of tumour. There is obvious importance in distinguishing between these two causes.

Radical radiotherapy typically causes tiredness and this is probably related to the volume of the brain requiring irradiation. That in turn is related to the size and location of the tumour, which may itself cause tiredness. Tiredness tends to accumulate during the course of treatment and may worsen for a short time after completion. Some patients recover early after radiotherapy, whilst in others a profound tiredness or somnolence may occur 4–6 weeks after radiotherapy. Pure acute somnolence is quite uncommon after cranial radiotherapy in adults. It is much more common following whole-brain radiotherapy in children. It is manifest as a relatively sudden onset of profound sleepiness 4–6 weeks after completing radiotherapy. It is self-limiting, although it is usually treated with steroids, and resolves within 1 or 2 weeks. This true somnolence may be very difficult to distinguish from tiredness associated both with the condition and its treatment. In fact, it seems likely that a spectrum exists from severe tiredness and lethargy at one end, to pure somnolence at the other.[2] Early recurrence may be difficult to identify because of limitations in brain imaging. Radiotherapy itself produces oedema in and around high-grade gliomas, perhaps due to tumour cell killing. Oedema, however, may be an early indication of recurrence of tumour. The tumour itself may regress very slowly after treatment, so that early post-radiotherapy imaging cannot typically distinguish between tumour that is regressing following treatment, from tumour that is progressing despite treatment. In this situation, an interval of a few weeks will usually make the differential diagnosis clear, but during that period, patient and carers may be severely distressed.

General management issues

Management of patients with relapse

The management of relapsed glioma should be considered on a individual basis. There will be patients who remain extremely well and a few of these have no detectable neurological deficit at the time that recurrence is identified. Other patients may have suffered significant problems from the relapse but they can nevertheless continue to lead an active life. The final group of patients are those in whom recurrence produces serious neurological deficit and in whom quality of life is seriously degraded. Typically, patients descend this ladder of neurological disability, passing through each step as the tumour progresses.

In broad terms the management strategies are the same as those as at the time of initial presentation. Although treatment is always palliative, in patients who are extremely fit, a more 'radical' approach may be appropriate; in the second group, a more conventional palliative approach should be taken; and in the third group, supportive care should be recommended. In term of 'radical' treatment of relapse, a few patients benefit from second operations. Broadly, this may be helpful where significant mass effect is present and where the tumour occupies a part of the brain that can be safely resected, such as the pole of the non-dominant frontal or temporal lobe. Usually this produces rapid improvement in symptoms and, in general craniotomy, is a well-tolerated procedure. Very rarely, a tumour regrows rapidly into the operative cavity. It is presumed that in such cases the pre-operative growth rate is limited by mass effect reducing tumour perfusion; following craniotomy and debulking, the mass effect being relieved, perfusion can be re-established, the tumour nourished, and rapid growth made possible. Fortunately, this is rare, though it preludes rapid decline. It is more common to undertake palliative chemotherapy as the first treatment for relapse. Some details of the chemotherapy are shown in Table 1.6. Chemotherapy is often combined with dexamethasone, at least initially. One of the specific reasons for undertaking chemotherapy is that response in the tumour will allow a reduction in dexamethasone dose and a consequential reduction in the side-effects of that treatment. Often, the patient's neurological condition improves with dexamethasone and can be maintained provided there is a response to chemotherapy.

In rare cases, particularly where there has been a long disease-free interval and where the tumour is comparatively small, re-treatment with radiotherapy may be considered. The patient must be fit enough to tolerate the treatment and the tumour should be small enough to avoid the risk of serious long-term damage. This is an uncommon situation but re-treatments appear to benefit a specific minority of patients.

Where recurrence has produced a rapid and major decline in neurological condition, it is usually obvious to the patient's family or significant others that further treatment may be difficult. Some patients remain intellectually intact and can take part in this discussion, but others become confused as a part of the illness. It is important, in our view, to explain the limitations of treatment, including the 'lose–lose' problem of having treatment, noted above.

A major problem for patients with serious deficits is one of everyday care. Patients with hemiplegia, for example, are extremely difficult to nurse at home simply because of the difficulties in moving, transferring, and going to the lavatory. It may be necessary to help potential carers to understand this burden, and in particular to help them deal with feelings of responsibility and guilt about not undertaking the patient's care in the final phase of the illness. Involvement of the palliative and Macmillan services is very valuable here. The role of hospice units is crucial in the management of patients with relapsed brain tumours. Relative under-provision in many parts of the country is distressing to all concerned, including hospice staff. It is important that prediction of survival time is difficult and unreliable, as the population survival curves in Figs 1.4–1.6 show. Thus, some patients who are expected to die quickly may linger for weeks or months, yet others who would seem ideally suited to hospice care may decline rapidly before transfer is possible.

In describing the outlook to patients and their families, some phrases are particularly helpful in describing possible prognosis. Although there is such large and unpredictable variation in individual survival, some generalizations are nevertheless usually possible. In the worst situation, the outlook may be 'days to weeks', if a little better 'weeks to months', and sometimes 'months to years'. This way of describing outlook avoids quoting a specific time-frame. Use of a numerical figure can be quite difficult psychologically for the patient, especially as the 'deadline' approaches. It also guards slightly against the inevitable error in predicting outcome.

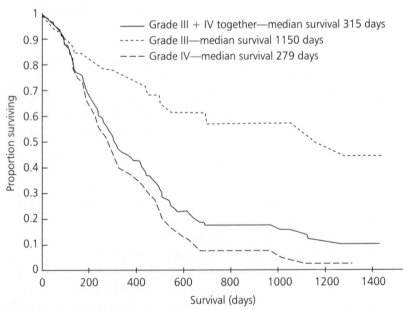

Fig. 1.4 Kaplan–Meier survival curves for patients with high-grade glioma (HGG) treated radically in our unit, distinguishing grade III from grade IV patients. The outcome is substantially different. Note that even amongst patients with grade IV tumours there is a small but important survival rate at 3 years (approximately 1100 days). Initial treatment is with radical radiotherapy, and on relapse, further treatment is offered to suitable patients, typically using chemotherapy. The term 'radical' means 'with curative intent'.

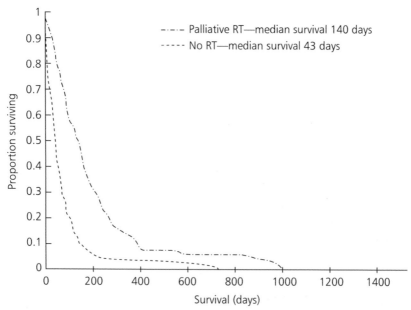

Fig. 1.5 Kaplan–Meier survival curves for patients with HGG treated in our unit with palliative radiotherapy or supportive care. Note the 'tail' on the two curves, due to surprisingly long survival in a few patients. This makes reliable prediction of outcome difficult.

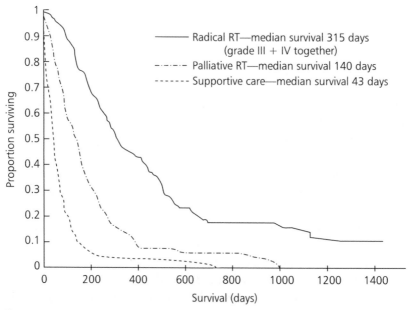

Fig. 1.6 Survival curves for HGG patients, comparing radical treatment (grade III and IV combined) with palliative radiotherapy and supportive care alone.

Outcome of patients receiving palliative radiotherapy

A small prospective study carried out in our unit between 1998 and 2000 reviewed 40 patients treated with palliative radiotherapy; 75% were either stable or improved after treatment, and in the majority, side-effects were minimal. In the 25% who deteriorated, the decline was not necessarily the result of the radiotherapy, but appeared to be due to progression of tumour despite treatment. The majority (25/40) of this group had a performance status of II or worse at referral. Their mean (not median) survival, from referral to oncology, was about 10 weeks, whilst for those with a better performance status, mean survival was 32 weeks. Patients with better performance status had a higher chance of responding, and those who had a neurological improvement had a longer survival. Note that these figures are for mean, not median survival.

These results show how important performance status is in predicting outcome, and also suggest that supportive care may be a reasonable alternative for patients whose neurological deficit gives them a poor performance status.

The patient pathway from presentation to death

High-grade gliomas present some of the most challenging problems in adult oncology and palliative care. One of the most distressing issues is that many tumours are able to resist the effects of treatment, or re-grow with comparative rapidity after treatment. A different way of looking at this problem is that gliomas are particularly resistant to radiotherapy and indeed to chemotherapy. In terms of curing tumours with these two modalities, every single cell in the tumour must be destroyed before the tumour can be cured. The unfortunate truth is that the current treatments are unable to kill sufficient cells to cure gliomas in all but the tiniest minority of patients, who presumably have unusually sensitive tumour cells. Treatment can however delay the progression of neurological deficit and, in a few patients, produce surprisingly long survival (see Fig. 1.4).

Discussions about survival overlook the important fact that once treatment ceases to be effective there is a period of life where quality of life and neurological function are often very poor. This is difficult to quantify because of difficulties in defining recurrence, in measuring neurological function and quality of life, and because patients may stop coming to hospital clinics. We studied a small group of 15 patients in whom the time to first recurrence was confirmed by CT or MRI imaging and in whom we also had date of death details. This group of patients is slightly selected, with a better outlook, because they were well enough to have recurrence confirmed by imaging. In this small group of 15 patients, the mean (not median) survival was 13 months, slightly better than average. However, the mean time from recurrence of tumour to death was actually 5 months, out of this 13-month period. This small group of patients were all treated radically and many would have been offered palliative chemotherapy on relapse, so that neurological function may not necessarily have declined immediately. However, this demonstrates that patients may be living with neurological deficits prior to death for a distressingly long period of time, representing a substantial proportion of their overall illness trajectory.

These considerations illustrate how important are further developments in treatment. Whilst there is no doubt that improvements that reduce side-effects are valuable, there would be an enormous social and personal benefit, if patients with high-grade gliomas could be offered some reasonable chance of cure.

Pituitary hormone dysfunction as a late side-effect of radiotherapy

Hormone dysfunction may occur due to the tumour itself and as a result of radiotherapy. Evidence from children suggests that most patients with primary brain tumours have hypothalamic-pituitary axis dysfunction at presentation. Similar evidence is not available for adults. Radiotherapy can affect hypothalamic–pituitary axis function, although usually there is a lag period of at least 1 or 2 years before this becomes manifest. For many patients with high-grade glioma this is not a practical consideration, but for patients with longer survival it is important. For example, in patients with low-grade glioma, in whom survival may be very long, this needs to be considered as part of routine follow-up, since it is unlikely that non-oncologists will focus on the issue. In assessing hypothalamic–pituitary axis function it is important for thyroid function tests to include free T4 levels. This may not be available in routine thyroid function tests in the community. If the hypothalamus is failing, it is possible for the patient to be hypothyroid, with a measured 'normal' TSH level but a low T4; the thyroid needs a higher level of stimulus to secrete the correct amount of thyroid hormone. Modern radiotherapy techniques of conformal radiotherapy offer an opportunity to reduce the dose delivered to the hypothalamus and pituitary, or reduce the number of patients in whom these structures are irradiated.

Shape of the glioma patient population survival curve

Population survival curves for patients with high-grade glioma show a curious biphasic shape, with an initial rapid decline in the proportion of patients surviving followed by a much shallower and surprisingly long tail (see Figs 1.4–1.6). These graphs show the survival for patients with HGG according to treatment intent, and it is telling that the basic shape of each curve is the same. The rapid initial part indicates the appalling outlook for many patients but the tail shows also the curious survival of a minority. This is presumed to relate to intrinsic factors within the tumour, which at present are not understood. Figure 1.6 suggests that delivering more treatment, i.e. a higher radiotherapy dose, affects both parts of the survival curve. The initial slope is made less steep and the second flatter slope is raised. This shape is mirrored in studies that have looked specifically at different radical radiotherapy doses, where a higher doses typically elevates both parts of the survival curve. This is important in considering future strategies because it suggests that *any* radiotherapy dose increase, provided that side-effects are no worse, would lead to a population benefit even if absolute cures were few.

Future strategies to improve treatment for patients with glioma

Improving tumour control

It seems extremely likely that a multi-modality approach will be required if we are to make a substantial impact on this disease. It is also important that modest improvements should deliver benefit in terms of lengthened survival to many patients, even if only a minority reach the 'tail' on the survival curve. Modern radiotherapy techniques such as conformal radiotherapy, or possibly intensity-modulated radiotherapy, may allow doses to be increased without a rise in the side-effects. This should mean that both parts of the population survival curve are improved, although modest dose increases are unlikely to cure many more patients.

Chemotherapy schedules at the moment are disappointing and new drugs are urgently needed. Possible developments include new drugs developed for new targets, specific to gliomas. Gene therapy has been investigated on a limited scale. It is encouraging that the virus vectors appear safe but, as yet, there is no convincing evidence that gene therapy alters outcome.

A curiosity in radiotherapy has been the discovery that rather low doses of radiation can produce as much tumour-cell kill as standard doses of the size used for each radiotherapy fraction. Radiotherapy schedules are currently being considered that might capitalize on this phenomenon. Unfortunately, treatment will have to be given three or four times per day, so this will be applicable to limited numbers of patients. Whether this strategy can be developed into a practical clinical schedule remains to be seen.

Reduction of side-effects of treatment

An equally important issue for patients with these conditions is the one of complications from treatment. It is important to refine our treatment techniques so as to improve the therapeutic ratio. New concepts with conformal therapy are helping to do this with patients receiving radical treatment. However, it seems likely that more attention to careful selection of patients for different treatment strategies would be useful and a better understanding of active palliative treatment is needed. Careful attention to the details of anticonvulsant and steroid treatment is a vital part of care at all sections of the illness trajectory. New anticonvulsant drugs can play a useful part but should be monitored by an experienced neurologist. Patient information and support, with respect to dexamethasone doses, are also worth while, particularly with the view to minimizing dexamethasone dose and its consequent side-effects.

Palliative and supportive care

Despite potential future developments, it is likely that substantial numbers of patients with gliomas, especially HGG, will not be cured. For these people and their families, access to palliative and supportive care services will remain a crucial component of management. Palliative and support services should be integrated with active treatment programmes, and these should be available continuously from the beginning of the illness pathway, though the role of palliative care may fluctuate during the illness trajectory. More research is warranted into how to optimize active treatment within the context of palliation. Addressing the under-provision of palliative and support services would make a major contribution to the overall care of this patient population.

Dexamethasone in the management of gliomas

Dexamethasone is a vital component in the management of patients with malignant CNS tumours. Its use will be considered in the different parts of the patient's pathway. In most situations, an educated guess for an appropriate dose is followed by titration of the dose against the patients symptoms and signs, either up or down, depending on clinical circumstances. The lower the dexamethasone dose the better, in order to minimize side-effects (Table 1.7).

Presentation and surgery

Most patients require dexamethasone at the time of presentation to alleviate symptoms and improve neurological deficits quickly. For patients presenting urgently, it is typical to start dexamethasone 4 mg four times a day prior to transfer to the neurosurgical unit. This is also the standard dose used for

Table 1.7 Side-effects of corticosteroids with particular relevance in neuro-oncology

Gastro-intestinal	**dyspepsia and peptic ulcer** oesophageal ulceration and candidiasis pancreatitis
Musculoskeletal	**proximal myopathy** **muscle pain** osteoporosis avascular necrosis of bone (e.g. head of femur) tendon rupture
Endocrine	**weight gain** **increased appetite** **adrenal suppression** **hyperglycaemia (diabetes)** amenorrhoea increased susceptibility to infection (e.g. shingles)
Neuropsychiatric	**euphoria** **insomnia** **psychosis** depression aggravation of epilepsy
Ophthalmic	**change in refractive index of cornea** cataract
Other	**peripheral oedema** **acne** **striae** hirsutism skin atrophy bruising impaired healing

Notes:

1. The side-effects with particular importance are shown first in bold.

2. The complication of change in refractive index of the cornea, due to water accumulation in the cornea, is important because it changes the correct prescription for glasses. However, as the dexamethasone dose changes so does the refractive index, so it is difficult to correct this in a practical way until the patient stops the steroid.

3. Steroid psychosis is a rare complication, but is very difficult to manage in patients with brain tumours where the therapeutic effect of the steroid is necessary to control intra-cranial pressure or mass effect.

4. Although aggravation of epilepsy is listed as a complication of steroid treatment, in the context of brain tumours dexamethasone normally improves epilepsy control, by reduction in the peri-tumoural oedema.

5. These side-effects can be summarized as Cushing's syndrome.

6. See the British National Formulary (BNF) for further information.

patients peri-operatively, where it plays a vital role in controlling traumatic oedema. Where presentation is less acute, lower doses may be used, though the 'full' dose is still needed peri-operatively.

Post-operatively, the dose can be reduced quite quickly to begin with, then more cautiously. The exact schedule will depend on the degree of mass effect pre-operatively, the extent of surgical resection, and the patient's recovery. Some patients may be able to stop dexamethasone shortly after surgery, whilst others have to remain on quite high doses.

Dexamethasone during radiotherapy

Radiotherapy causes a modest increase in oedema, especially later in the course. This may be due to the secondary effects of tumour-cell kill, though this is not certain. Where little or no mass effect exists, the small increase in volume around a tumour can be accommodated, so that steroids may not be needed. Where significant intracranial mass effect is present, this small change cannot be accommodated and must be actively treated with steroid.

Dexamethasone is thus not necessary in all patients having radiotherapy for LGG or HGG. Those who do not need steroids when they start radiotherapy will usually complete treatment without, though this is relatively uncommon. Patients on a low dose when starting, for example 4 mg per day or less, may be able to reduce during radiotherapy. Patients requiring high doses usually cannot reduce at all.

Dexamethasone dose after radiotherapy

In patients who have had radical radiotherapy, the general strategy should be to reduce the dose once the acute side-effects have passed, with a view to stopping the drug altogether.

Moderate- to high-dose dexamethasone is the common situation in patients having palliative radiotherapy. In these patients, about three-quarters stabilize or improve following radiotherapy, and a quarter deteriorate. For the majority it is unwise to reduce the steroid dose on completing radiotherapy. A better strategy is to review the situation after 4–6 weeks. If the patient is thriving, then a dose reduction is indicated. If not, then either the dose should be maintained or increased.

Strategy for dose reduction

Just how fast a dose reduction can be accomplished depends on the dose and its duration. Usually, the patient with a CNS tumour has been on dexamethasone for several months before it is possible to attempt withdrawal. In these circumstances the usual strategy is:

to reach 4 mg per day—reduce by 2 mg (per day) each fortnight;

from 4 to 2 mg per day—reduce by 1 mg (per day) each fortnight;

from 2 to 0.5 mg per day—reduce by 0.5 mg (per day) each fortnight;

from 0.5 mg per day—reduce to 0.5 mg on alternate days, then stop.

The final steps are smaller, since part of the function of gentle withdrawal is to allow the hypothalamic–pituitary-adrenal axis to recover its function. Since normal adrenal steroid production is equivalent to approximately 0.75 mg of dexamethasone per day, the final steps are actually quite large in physiological terms. A few patients who have been on steroids for a very long time are unable to tolerate even these steps. In such cases, a change to the equivalent dose of prednisolone is worthwhile because smaller, slower steps can be taken, at the rate of 1 mg (per day) per month (see Table 1.8).

A few patients with high-grade gliomas appear unable to stop steroids whatever strategy is employed. It may be more compassionate and pragmatic to minimize the dose without necessarily coming into conflict with the patient in repeated attempts to stop.

The patient, and primary carer, should be advised that if a significant deterioration occurs, over and above tiredness lasting a few days, then the previous dose should be re-instituted, and the programme reviewed.

Strategy for dose increase at the time of relapse

Dexamethasone is a valuable treatment at the time of relapse. Quite often, patients experience a surprisingly sudden decline in neurological function as

Table 1.8 Equivalent doses of dexamethasone

Dexamethasone	0.75 mg
Hydrocortisone	20 mg
Prednisolone	5 mg

Notes:

1. The physiological production of corticosteroids amounts to the equivalent of dexamethasone of about 0.75–1.13 mg per day (hydrocortisone 20–30 mg).

2. If a patient has difficulty coming off dexamethasone completely it may be helpful to change to the equivalent dose of prednisolone, which can be reduced in smaller steps, and at a slower rate such as 1 mg per month.

3. It is worth considering whether the hypothalamic–pituitary axis may have been damaged by the tumour or treatment. In occasional patients this complicates steroid withdrawal and needs specialist endocrinological input.

4. See the British National Formulary (BNF) for further information.

recurrence occurs. Presumably the tumour can re-grow without causing further deficit until a critical point is suddenly reached, akin to the 'straw breaking the camel's back'. At this point dexamethasone treatment is usually implemented.

The dose to use depends on the severity of the deficit that has occurred and on its impact on the patient's life. If this is severe, then a dose of 16 mg per day, as 4 mg four times daily or 8 mg twice daily, is appropriate. If the deficit is modest, then a proportionately lower dose can be used, such as 4 mg twice daily. Occasionally, the deficit appears more slowly, especially in a patient with recurrent LGG, so that it is less severe when the patient re-presents. In this case, a smaller dose such as 2 mg twice daily can be used, while the patient is investigated.

Stopping dexamethasone as a therapeutic strategy

At the end of the illness trajectory, when the patient is no longer awake, and particularly if side-effects of protracted dexamethasone administration become serious, it may be an appropriate strategy to consider acute withdrawal of the steroids. In our experience this should always be done in consultation with the family or significant others. A clear explanation seeking agreement is usually reassuring that the medical and nursing teams have the best interests of the patient uppermost, whereas undertaking this strategy without consultation may give the impression of an underhand approach with a hidden agenda. This strategy is often kindly. However, occasionally the expected outcome of rapid deterioration does not occur immediately, which can be distressing to all concerned. Being aware that this does occasionally happen can provide some reassurance.

Dexamethasone and anticonvulsants

Both phenytoin and carbamazepine increase the liver metabolism of dexamethasone through the cytochrome P450 pathway. In effect this means that the effective circulating drug levels may be lower than the nominal dose suggests. It may be appropriate to give higher doses than the lists above suggest, in these circumstances. However, in the end, the dose should be titrated against the patients symptoms and signs.

Acknowledgements

We are grateful to many palliative medicine doctors and nurses, who, over the years, have helped us to understand how to integrate our specialties for the benefit of our patients, but in particular Drs Sara Booth, Michael Minton,

Janet Squire, and Professor Ilora Finlay. We also thank Mrs Jane Sales and Mrs Carol Moxey for their help with the preparation of the manuscript, and to Mrs Lorraine Muffett and Miss Kate Burton for helpful suggestions and comments.

References

1   Do, V., Gebski, V., and Barton, M. B. (2000) .The effect of waiting for radiotherapy for grade III/IV gliomas. *Radiother Oncol* **57**(2), 131–6.

2   Faithfull, S. and Brada, M. (1998). Somnolence syndrome in adults following cranial irradiation for primary brain tumours. *Clin Oncol* **10**(4), 250–4.

Further reading

Davies, E. and Hopkins, A. (ed.) (1997). *Improving care for patients with malignant cerebral glioma.* Royal College of Physicians of London, London.

Guerrero, D. (ed.) (1998). *Neuro-oncology for nurses.* Whurr Publishers, London.

Medical Research Council Brain Tumour Working Party (1990). Prognostic factors for high-grade malignant glioma: development of a prognostic index. Report of the Medical Research Council Brain Tumour Working Party. *J Neurooncol* **9**(1), 47–55.

Nieder, C., Grosu, A. L., and Molls, M. (2000). A comparison of treatment results for recurrent malignant gliomas. *Cancer Treat Rev* **26**(6), 397–409.

Chapter 2

Management of patients with brain metastasis

Vinay K. Puduvalli and Terri S. Armstrong

Introduction

The detection of brain metastasis in patients with cancer signals a dire turn in the course of the disease. These patients often have fewer treatment options, a poorer quality of life, and an abbreviated lifespan. Often, the diagnosis of brain metastasis in the course of aggressive therapy for systemic cancer may change the direction of management toward palliative care because of the poor prognosis associated with this finding. There is an increasing awareness of the unmet needs of patients with advanced cancer, including those who have metastatic disease. Additionally, it has been recognized that many patients fail to receive the full benefit of such care, as they reach the terminal stages of the disease. This has fuelled interest in studies directed toward a better understanding of the disease process, its natural history, modification by therapy, and end-of-life issues associated with brain metastasis. This chapter presents an overview of treatment strategies for patients with brain metastasis and reviews the factors to be considered in the optimal management of these patients. These guidelines are derived from large controlled studies, where such data are available. However, because of a paucity of studies regarding certain aspects of the disease, guidelines in these instances are derived from smaller case series or from guidelines for standards of care published by national medical organizations, which in turn have formulated them on the basis of a consensus of opinion among the experts in the fields and from cumulative evidence from various studies.

Brain metastases are the most common intra-cranial tumours, outnumbering primary brain tumours nearly 10-fold. With the exception of metastases from small cell lung cancer (SCLC), it occurs in advanced stages of cancer, often with widespread systemic metastasis and in patients who have failed multiple therapies. Various types of cancer metastasize to the brain with strikingly different frequencies related both to the incidence of the primary

Table 2.1 Distribution of cancer types among patients with brain metastasis

Type of cancer	%
Lung cancer	34
Breast cancer	21
Melanoma	12
Renal cancer	8
Gastro-intestinal cancer	6
Other	19

cancer and to its biological propensity to metastasize to this organ system (Table 2.1). The primary cancers most commonly associated with brain metastasis are lung cancer, breast cancer, melanoma, renal cancer, and colon cancer. Even within a histologic type, some subtypes of cancer, such as SCLC or lung adenocarcinoma, have a higher predilection for metastasizing to the brain, probably because of their biological characteristics. In these subtypes, brain metastasis not only can occur early in the disease but also can be the presenting feature of these malignancies, leading to further workup and subsequent detection of the primary.

Most brain metastases (~80%) are supratentorial, and nearly 50% are multiple. Melanomas, lung cancer, and breast cancer commonly present with multiple metastases, whereas others such as renal cancer, usually result in single lesions. Younger patients are more likely to develop brain metastasis even after adjusting for their longer survival. This may be due to biological factors specific to this age group. The systemic disease burden may independently affect the patient's functional status. Additionally, the neurological symptoms that accompany brain metastasis can significantly add to clinical morbidity, worsening an already compromised quality of life in these patients. Hence, along with therapeutic measures aimed at controlling the disease when appropriate, optimal management of neurological symptoms concurrent with other palliative measures should be an essential component of the treatment plan; this can greatly help optimize quality of life for these patients in the face of advancing disease.

For the purpose of formulating a rational approach to therapy, the management of patients with brain metastasis can be conveniently viewed as having two components: oncological (treatment of the malignant metastasis) and neurological (management of the clinical manifestations of nervous system involvement), although it should be recognized that these are inseparable aspects of a single disease process. The following sections will address the issues that affect clinical decision-making, using these components as guidelines.

Brain metastasis—diagnostic and therapeutic strategies

Initial management

Brain metastasis in patients with systemic malignancy is usually diagnosed either because of the development of neurological symptoms or after a routine radiological assessment for screening purposes. The neurological presentation can be either diffuse (including symptoms such as encephalopathy, progressive cognitive changes, and global headache) or focal (including limb weakness, sensory disturbances, focal or secondary generalized seizures, language disturbance, and visual deficits), as summarized in Table 2.2. If patients are lethargic or obtunded due to intra-cranial disease, as revealed by focal deficits preceding an alteration in mental status, papilloedema, or a history of brain metastasis, aggressive management of oedema with steroids or other anti-oedema measures, including osmotic agents, hyperventilation, and diuretics, may be indicated in patients who are not considered to be in the terminal stages of their disease and have a reasonable expectation for continued survival and treatment. It should be recognized that encephalopathy can also result from non-convulsive status epilepticus, a condition that can be identified by electro-encephalography (EEG) recording and should be managed using intravenous anticonvulsants with close monitoring. Hydrocephalus resulting from an obstructive lesion can also cause progressive alteration of consciousness that may require immediate surgical intervention, regardless of whether the culprit lesion is a single metastasis or one of multiple brain lesions. Lastly, the routine rules of the emergency management of seriously compromised patients including evaluation of airway, respiration, and cardiovascular function, are

Table 2.2 Signs and symptoms associated with brain metastasis

Symptoms		Signs	
Headache	49%	Hemiparesis	59%
Altered mental status	32%	Impaired cognitive function	58%
Focal weakness	30%	Hemisensory loss	21%
Ataxia	21%	Papilloedema	20%
Seizures	18%	Ataxia	19%
Speech difficulty	12%	Aphasia	18%

also applicable. Some of these issues are dealt with in greater detail in other chapters of this volume. Once the patient's condition is stabilized, the workup to determine the further course of treatment, should include an assessment of the number and locations of intra-cranial lesions, the extent of systemic disease, and the functional status of the patient.

Diagnostic issues

The number and locations of brain metastases are critical factors in determining approaches to treatment, independent of the histologic subtype. This can best be determined with a magnetic resonance imaging (MRI) scan with contrast enhancement, which is hence recommended as the imaging of choice whenever it can be obtained. The ability to pick up small lesions has improved with the use of triple-dose contrast-enhanced MRI. Supratentorial single, enhancing lesions are metastatic tumours in ~90% of patients with known cancer. This frequency is even higher in patients who have multiple enhancing lesions. In these cases, surgery for diagnostic purposes is usually not required for treatment planning. However, patients who present with enhancing brain lesions but do not yet have a diagnosis of cancer need a diagnostic workup to ascertain if the lesions are a result of a disease process unrelated to cancer or to detect the primary malignancy and determine the extent of systemic disease. This may detect other lesions that are more easily accessible for diagnostic surgical sampling. This approach also has a therapeutic advantage; for instance, if a radiosensitive tumour is detected by bronchoscopy and biopsy, the patient could proceed to whole brain radiation therapy (WBRT) without having to be subjected to a craniotomy.

It is important to bear in mind that other disease processes can result in single or multiple enhancing brain lesions in patients with cancer, although this is relatively uncommon. Other lesions in the brain can result from abscesses, demyelinating processes, cerebrovascular events (ischaemic or haemorrhagic), primary brain tumours, or radiation necrosis. Patients with cancer may be immunocompromised by their malignancy or by treatments such as steroids or chemotherapy. This may enable opportunistic infections to occur, sometimes without florid signs of infection, which would pose a diagnostic dilemma. In such cases, the presence of a known systemic infection, low-grade fevers, signs and symptoms of meningeal irritation, the radiological finding of ring-enhancing lesions with thin uniform walls and oedema, or a history of exposures or prior illnesses may alert the vigilant clinician to the possibility of an infectious aetiology for such lesions. In some instances, only a resection of the mass may enable the diagnosis. Enhancing lesions may also result from radiation injury or radiation-induced secondary neoplasms in patients who have previously been irradiated for metastatic brain disease or skull base disease. Although these aetiologies are uncommon, the correct diagnosis of such non-metastatic lesions would clearly prompt a different therapeutic approach than would be used for brain metastasis.

Therapeutic approaches

The optimal therapeutic approach for brain metastasis is determined by several variables, which should be carefully considered in each patient (Table 2.3). The most important of these variables are the systemic disease burden and the neurological and functional status of the patient at presentation. Given that brain metastasis occurs mostly in the setting of advanced cancer, treatment selection should be based on reasonable evidence of benefit; such treatment should be tailored to the functional status of the patient and the extent of systemic disease, which may determine the outcome independent of the brain disease. In fact, patients with brain metastasis more commonly die from progression of their systemic disease rather than from neurological causes. Hence, the expectations of the patient and the physician regarding the outcome of therapy should be discussed at length and clearly outlined before beginning treatment. These discussions ideally should address issues such as expectations regarding the amelioration of neurological deficits, the estimated duration of such benefits, the effect of treatment on quality of life and survival, and the potentially palliative nature of the therapy in the face of aggressive disease. However, the scarcity of data regarding these issues may make it

Table 2.3 Factors to be considered in management of patients with brain metastases

Patient and cancer factors
Age
Overall functional status
Neurological deficits
Status of systemic cancer
Brain metastasis factors
Number
Size
Locations
Co-morbid conditions
Leptomeningeal spread
Hydrocephalus
Seizures
Depression

Table 2.4 Guidelines for management of patients with brain metastasis

Organization	Nomenclature	World Wide Web address
National Comprehensive Cancer Network	Practice guidelines	www.nccn.org
American College of Radiology	Appropriateness criteria	www.acr.org/dyna/?id = appropriateness_criteria
Cancer Care Ontario Practice guidelines Initiative	Practice guidelines (in development)	www.ccopebc.ca/guidelines.html

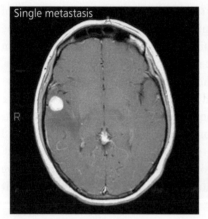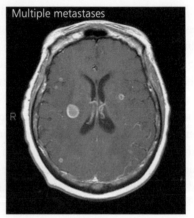

Fig. 2.1 MRI scan showing a single right temporal metastasis (left) and multiple bilateral metastases (right).

difficult for physicians and patients alike to make decisions and predict the course of the disease in response to a given treatment. Consensus guidelines for the management of patients with brain metastasis have been developed by several organizations, and the reader is referred to these guidelines for further information on this subject (Table 2.4).

The decision-making process for patients with brain metastasis usually starts with the onset of a neurological event, followed by evaluation with an imaging study that reveals the brain lesion. The detection of single or multiple lesions thus becomes the first fork in the decision tree that is subsequently utilized to determine optimal management. Hence, this is used as a guideline for examining the management of these patients for the purpose of this chapter (Fig. 2.1).

Management of patients with single brain metastases

At the outset, it is important for the clinician to recognize the difference between a single brain metastases (which is a single brain lesion in the presence of other systemic metastases) and a solitary metastasis (which is the only metastatic lesion in the body). The initial management of patients who have a single metastasis, confirmed by an MRI scan of adequate quality, is to determine the systemic disease burden and the patients' overall functional status. Patients who have limited or absent systemic disease and a good functional status are generally good candidates for further treatment of brain metastases. Treatment modalities that are used include WBRT, surgery, stereotactic radiosurgery (SRS), or various combinations of these modalities (Fig. 2.2). Chemotherapy does not have a defined role in the management of these patients. Despite various studies, however, the optimal management of patients with single brain metastases remains to be established.

Because of certain limitations in the use of local therapy and the lack of evidence of benefit in these patients until recently, the recommended therapy for all patients with single brain metastases had been WBRT. This was based on the results of several studies conducted by the Radiation Therapy Oncology Group (RTOG) and others that tested the efficacy of various RT dosages and schedules. For example, a dose-response effect was seen in a randomized trial (RTOG 85–28) of hyperfractionated WBRT for patients with unresected brain metastases that enrolled 153 patients with solitary metastases with higher doses of WBRT proving superior in improving survival.[1] Improvement in neurological function was also seen with higher doses but did not reach statistical significance. Favourable prognostic factors included age <60 years, a Karnofsky Performance Score (KPS) >90, controlled primary cancer, and

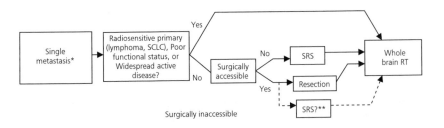

*Patients with no known cancer and a single lesion suggestive of a metastatic lesion on an MRI scan will require a workup for detecting a primary malignancy.
**Based on preliminary reports, SRS may potentially be as effective as surgery in resectable single metastases but this approach has the disadvantage that a histologic diagnosis cannot be obtained.

Fig. 2.2 Management of patients with single-brain metastasis.

the absence of other systemic metastases. Several other studies have indicated that WBRT is beneficial in treating patients with single metastases.

With improvements in radiological and surgical techniques, the role of surgery was subsequently assessed in other controlled trials, investigating whether surgery alone, WBRT alone, or surgery followed by WBRT was the most beneficial to patients with single brain metastases. In a randomized trial of patients with single brain metastases, patients received either WBRT or surgery followed by WBRT. The combination of surgery and WBRT proved better than WBRT alone in terms of increasing survival, decreasing the rate of recurrence, and improving quality of life. This was also seen in a separate randomized study reported on by Noordijk et al.,[2] in which patients were enrolled into WBRT alone or surgery plus WBRT. The latter group had a longer survival and showed a trend toward longer functionally independent survival.

The related question of whether surgery alone would suffice for these patients was investigated in subsequent trials. In a randomized, multicentre trial of patients with single metastases who underwent gross total resection alone or followed by WBRT, Patchell et al.[3] observed that post-operative RT, as opposed to surgery alone, appeared to decrease the frequency of recurrence both at the original site and in other parts of the brain (the primary endpoint of this study) and to reduce the likelihood of the patient dying of neurological causes. However, the overall survival and the length of time patients were functionally independent were the same in the two groups. Overall, the results of these studies can be interpreted to mean that people with single metastatic brain lesions should be treated with gross total resection plus WBRT when feasible. The reader is referred to an excellent review of some of these studies by Weinberg and colleagues.[4] Although no survival advantage is apparent in these studies, there is evidence that function is better preserved and the burden of brain disease is decreased by this approach. It could also be postulated that in the future, if the rate of death from neurological causes surpasses that from systemic causes in these patients (for instance, because of better control of systemic cancer), gains in survival may also be expected.

The role of radiosurgery in patients with single brain metastases has been of great interest because it could offer a non-invasive alternative to surgery and can be used to treat surgically inaccessible lesions. However, there have been no randomized prospective studies comparing radiosurgery and surgery for single brain metastases. There have also been no randomized studies comparing radiosurgery plus WBRT with surgery plus WBRT. The results of such studies will be of obvious importance in guiding therapy in the future. Selected patients with a poor functional status or with a surgically inaccessible lesion who are not candidates for surgery may derive the benefit of aggressive local therapy through radiosurgery. In a retrospective study, Shirato *et al.*[5] determined the effect of SRS alone without WBRT in 44 patients with single brain metastases and reported a median survival of 8.5 months with a 1-year survival of 34%. Additionally, in a multicentre retrospective study of 122 patients with single brain metastases treated with SRS plus WBRT, Auchter *et al.*[6] observed an actuarial median survival of 56 weeks with a 1-year survival rate of 53%. On the basis of these results, the authors suggested that SRS might be able to replace surgery as a primary treatment modality, citing the advantages that it is non-invasive and cost-effective, that morbidity is reduced, and that it has a wider application than surgery. In an interesting addendum to this issue, cost analysis done by the same group studying patients with single metastases treated with surgery versus those treated with SRS showed that surgery resulted in a 1.8-fold higher cost than SRS. A few studies have also shown the usefulness of SRS in treating brainstem metastases that are otherwise not accessible to surgery. The reader is referred to a detailed review of the results of some of these studies and their implications by Flickinger.[7] These reports strongly suggest that radiosurgery may prove to be an effective, non-invasive alternative to surgery in the treatment of patients with single metastases and may be cost-effective. These results remain to be proven in prospective studies, which are currently ongoing.

It is important for the clinician to recognize that there were important patient selection criteria applied in the controlled studies described above. For example, in the study examining the role of surgery in this population, patients with a KPS <70, those with leptomeningeal disease, patients requiring urgent therapy, and those with radiosensitive primary tumours, such as SCLC, germ cell tumours, lymphoma, leukaemia, or multiple myeloma, were excluded from the study. Thus, patients with highly radiosensitive tumours may be better served by using WBRT first and, if the lesions recur after such therapy and systemic disease remains stable, local therapies such as surgery or radiosurgery should be considered. The results of such studies should, therefore, be interpreted judiciously when these treatments are considered in patients who do not fulfil the criteria set in such studies; it is the clinician's responsibility to appropriately interpret the conclusions reached in these studies when applying them to a given patient.

Management of patients with multiple brain metastases

There are limited treatment options for patients with multiple brain metastases and these are generally palliative in nature (Fig. 2.3). Studies conducted by the RTOG and other groups have shown that WBRT is effective in these patients. This approach is based on the rationale that WBRT targets not only

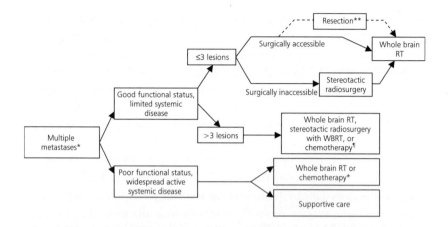

*Patients with no known cancer and multiple lesions suggestive of metastases of an MRI scan will require a workup for detecting a primary malignancy. If no other surgically accessible lesions are noted, the brain lesions should be targets of biopsy or resection.
**Selected patients may be eligible for surgical resection of multiple accessible lesions before WBRT. Additionally, symptomatic lesions may need to be resected prior to WBRT.
¶Chemotherapy is usually reserved for patients who have chemosensitive tumors.

Fig. 2.3 Management of patients with multiple-brain metastases.

the multiple lesions seen on imaging studies, but also those that may be microscopic and not evident on radiological studies. The RTOG conducted several studies evaluating the role of WBRT in an attempt to find an optimal dose and schedule. These studies showed that WBRT could be palliative in patients with multiple metastases (Fig. 2.4).[8] The term multiple brain metastases has been variably used to describe lesions varying from 2 to >50. However, >80% of patients with brain metastases harbour 1–4 lesions. Recognizing this fact, studies have been conducted to reassess the role of local therapy in patients who have 1–4 lesions.

Better radiological definition of the extent and number of lesions and improvements in surgical techniques in recent years have helped investigators reassess the role of local therapies in the treatment of multiple brain metastases. Such local therapies include radiosurgery and surgical resection. Interstitial radiation has also been studied, but the role of this approach is considered limited at present.

Radiosurgery has also been used to treat multiple address several lesions, often with subsequent WBRT. Kondziolka *et al.*[9] conducted a randomized trial in which patients with 2–4 metastatic brain lesions received either WBRT alone or SRS plus WBRT. Local failure was seen in all patients who received WBRT alone, but in only 8% of patients with SRS plus WBRT. Median time to local failure was 6 months with WBRT alone and 36 months with SRS plus

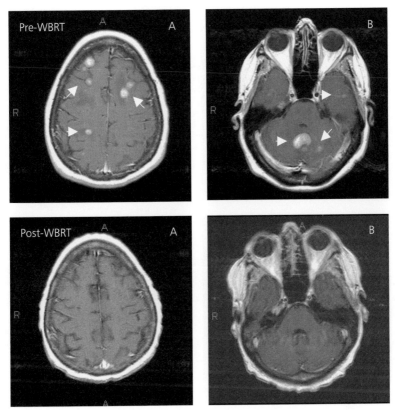

Fig. 2.4 MRI scan showing dramatic response of multiple brain metastases to WBRT in a 56-year-old caucasian female with metastatic breast cancer.

WBRT. Further, a trend toward increased median survival was seen in the group receiving SRS plus WBRT, but it did not reach statistical significance. Other studies (mostly retrospective or non-randomized) have shown similar results.[6,8] A phase-III RTOG study (RTOG 9508) evaluating WBRT alone (37.5 Gy in 15 fractions) versus radiosurgery (15–24 Gy) plus WBRT in patients with 1–3 lesions is currently ongoing. Another ongoing study conducted by the European Organization for Research and Treatment of Cancer (EORTC) is comparing patients receiving SRS alone (20 Gy) with those receiving SRS followed by WBRT (30 Gy in 10 fractions).

When patients present with large tumours or lesions that produce neurological symptoms, surgery should be considered to decrease the immediate morbidity before radiation therapy is started. For example, recent studies have suggested that, in carefully selected patients, it is feasible to resect several accessible metastatic lesions in the same surgical session, with the resultant patient survival

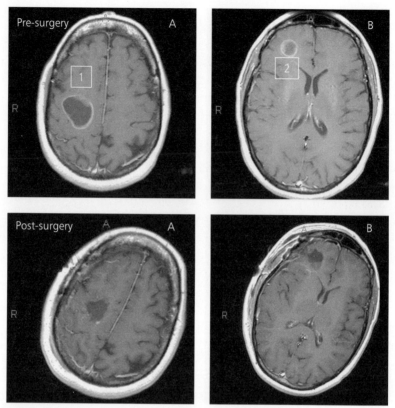

Fig. 2.5 MRI scan showing resection of two accessible metastatic brain lesions in a single surgical procedure.

similar to that achieved in patients with single resectable lesions (Fig. 2.5).[10] However, questions regarding which local therapy is optimal remain to be examined prospectively. For example, the controversy over the benefit of radio-surgery versus surgery in patients with multiple metastases needs to be settled. Bindal *et al.*,[10] however, who reported the results of a retrospective study, observed that patients who undergo surgery appear to have a longer survival and a better quality of life than those who undergo radiosurgery alone. They therefore concluded that radiosurgery should be reserved for patients who cannot undergo surgery.

Management of patients with recurrent brain metastases

The optimal management of recurrent lesions in patients who have had surgery or radiation therapy is uncertain. Most of these patients will have widely metastatic or advanced primary disease that precludes further aggressive therapy. When patients have become debilitated from their systemic disease burden and are recognized as poor candidates for further treatment of their malignancy, the focus should be on symptom control and palliative care, which is often most appropriately administered in a hospice setting. A minority of patients may develop recurrent brain disease and have no active systemic disease. In these patients, treatment planning involves evaluation of the number, locations, and sizes of the metastases. Accessible single lesions that are associated with neurological symptoms because of oedema may be amenable to resection. Those that are inaccessible to surgery or are close to eloquent areas of the brain may be treatable with radiosurgery. Selected patients who were previously treated with WBRT and have recurrent disease may benefit from SRS, as reported by Shaw et al.[11] in one study (RTOG 90–05). Patients who were previously treated with surgery or radiosurgery alone, and have recurrence in distant brain sites, may be candidates for WBRT. However, the impact of such interventions on survival is not well established; therefore, careful patient selection is critical in making such decisions. Good functional status and younger age are favourable prognostic factors. Studies of this aspect of the disease will be particularly relevant as better therapies are developed for the primary malignancies and patients live longer, exposing them to an increased risk of both initial and recurrent brain metastasis.

Role of chemotherapy in treatment of brain metastases

Patients with brain metastasis have generally been considered poor candidates for chemotherapy because of several factors, including the possibility of systemic side-effects that may compromise quality of life, the resistance of most tumour histological types to chemotherapies, and issues regarding the blood–brain barrier. However, it has also been recognized that a subgroup of patients, particularly those with small cell lung cancer or breast cancer, may indeed respond well to chemotherapy. In a phase-III study conducted by the EORTC in patients with SCLC with brain metastasis, the combination of teniposide and WBRT resulted in significantly higher response rates and a longer time to progression but did not translate into an increased survival compared with WBRT alone.[12] In a randomized study, Twelves et al.[13] observed a response rate of 53% in 19 patients who received chemotherapy alone for brain metastasis from SCLC. They therefore recommended a re-evaluation of the role of chemotherapy in chemo-sensitive tumours such as SCLC. This recommendation was also made by Bernardo et al.,[14] who reported an overall response rate of 45% in 20 evaluable patients with non-small-cell lung cancer (NSCLC) with a median duration of response of 25 weeks. Recent studies have also shown the potential efficacy of newer chemotherapy agents such as temozolomide, alone or in combination with WBRT or other agents, in this setting. Because of its relatively better toxicity profile and the ease of oral administration, temozolomide may be particularly useful in patients with brain metastasis and advanced systemic disease in terms of better preserving of quality of life. In a randomized phase-II trial comparing temozolomide plus WBRT with WBRT alone, treatment with temozolomide was associated with a greater response rate (96% vs. 67%) and improvement in neurological function.[15] The combination of temozolomide and thalidomide has recently been shown to have activity, even in a recalcitrant tumour subtype, such as a brain metastasis from melanoma.[16] Despite these early results, large studies in selected patient populations are necessary before the role of chemotherapy in these patients can be established. With the advent of newer therapies that cross the blood–brain barrier and have activity against the primary tumour, an expanded role for chemotherapy may be anticipated in the future.

Prognostic factors in patients with brain metastases

Using recursive partitioning analysis (RPA), Gaspar *et al.*[17] analysed data from three phase-III trials, conducted by the RTOG in patients with brain metastasis evaluating WBRT, to determine prognostic factors that affected patient outcome. Based on their findings from this analysis, they proposed three prognostic groups: RPA class I—patients with KPS $\geq$ 70, under 65 years of age, with controlled primary and no extra-cranial metastases; RPA class III—KPS <70; RPA class II—all others. This has been validated in other trials showing that patients in RPA class I are most likely to respond to aggressive therapy with a median survival of 7–12 months, and may be candidates for clinical trials. RPA class-II patients had a median survival of approximately 4 months. Additionally, retrospective analyses (despite their recognized potential for bias) have shown that the RPA classes may be valid for patients who receive treatment such as surgery plus WBRT or radiosurgery plus WBRT, and may guide the selection of patients for such treatments.

Management of neurological symptoms

The proper evaluation and optimal management of neurological symptoms is a major component of the therapeutic strategy for patients with brain metastasis, particularly with respect to maintaining quality of life. Common signs and symptoms that occur in people with brain metastasis are outlined in Table 2.2. The management of associated conditions, such as increased intra-cranial pressure, seizures, and neuropsychiatric symptoms, is presented in detail in other chapters in this volume. Other relevant symptoms that can disrupt the patient's quality of life are briefly outlined in the following sections.

Headache

Headache is the most common presenting symptom in people with metastatic brain tumours. It usually results from the disturbance of cranial pain-sensitive structures, such as the meninges, blood vessels, and cranial nerves. Headaches related to metastasis are most commonly worse in the morning and may awaken the patient during the night. Given that headaches are a common disorder in the general population, it is important to obtain a thorough history regarding the type, location, and intensity of the headache and any aggravating or relieving factors. For example, in a patient with known cancer and a long history of migraine headaches (typically throbbing unilateral headaches associated with nausea, photophobia or phonophobia, and sometimes preceded by auras or precipitated by dietary triggers), the occurrence of a dull non-throbbing unilateral headache without the characteristics that the patient may attribute to his/her typical headaches should alert the physician to the possibility of metastatic disease. If such headaches are accompanied by papilloedema, there is a high likelihood of brain metastasis.

A recent analysis by Christiaans and colleagues[18] revealed that intra-cranial metastases were found in 32.4% of the cancer patients with headache as the presenting symptom. Clinical predictors included headache duration <10 weeks, emesis, and pain not of tension type. However, these predictors had low specificity, and the authors recommended an MRI to evaluate all patients with a history of cancer who develop new-onset headache or experience a significant alteration from pre-existing headache. Treatment of headache usually requires relief of oedema and treatment of the lesion. Steroids provide short-term analgesia by decreasing vasogenic oedema. Studies have shown that up to 70% of patients with brain metastasis may improve clinically in response to steroids and experience increased survival times. Opioid and non-opioid analgesics may also be used as clinically appropriate. Steroids should not be used, however, when lymphoma is suspected, because steroids in this setting can rapidly induce apoptosis and cause a dramatic decrease in the tumour mass before biopsy, causing false-negative results. Once the immediate symptoms are addressed, a more sustained relief from symptoms can usually be achieved only through treatment of the lesions with surgical resection, radiation therapy, or chemotherapy.

Focal symptoms

The occurrence of focal neurological deficits strongly suggests a focal pathology in the nervous system and in systemic cancer, this is usually a result of due to brain metastasis. Similar to those of other lesions that can affect the brain, focal symptoms of brain metastasis depend on tumour location. A spectrum of deficits can occur, including language disturbances (such as including expressive and comprehensive aphasia), impairment of higher cognitive functions, loss of vision (hemianopsia or quadrantanopsia), hemiparesis, sensory disturbance, cranial neuropathies, and ataxia. Such overt symptoms and signs can easily bring attention to the nervous system involvement; however, patients occasionally harbour multiple metastases in both supratentorial and infratentorial compartments and manifest only subtle and non-focal symptoms that may fail to raise the possibility of brain metastases and may delay detection and treatment.

The management of deficits from brain metastasis depends on several factors. Focal deficits that are predominantly due to vasogenic oedema will often respond to steroid therapy. Those resulting from direct involvement of an eloquent area of the brain are likely to cause long-standing deficits. In either case, the use of steroids along with aggressive physical and occupational therapy is important in salvaging function in the short term. Concurrent treatment of the lesion when feasible will provide more longstanding improvement if the treatment contains the disease process. Speech therapy should be considered for deficits related to language. The involvement of rehabilitative services for a comprehensive evaluation and an assessment of the patients' functional needs in their own environment are critical in providing meaningful support to patients neurologically disabled from their brain metastasis.

Measures to identify and address issues regarding safety

Safety is an issue for patients with all levels of physical and cognitive impairment related to brain metastasis, both at home and during inpatient treatment. Particular attention must be paid to ensure the safety of patients, even if they have subtle deficits. Formal neuropsychological evaluation allows a better characterization of cognitive deficits and identification of functional limitations, which in turn can assist in arranging a structured and safe environment for the patient and maximize their function. In patients with mild or circumscribed impairments, cognitive retraining may be effective, whereas other patients may benefit from the use of behavioural compensation techniques. Additional issues include safety measures and legal requirements in patients with seizures. If patients have had seizures, they should be made aware of the state or federal regulations regarding driving. In relevant cases, rehabilitation facilities also offer formalized driving evaluations to ascertain difficulties people may have in a simulated driving environment.

Symptom management at the end of life

The management of symptoms at the end of life is critical both for both the comfort of the patient and for the family's peace of mind. As tumours grow within the cranial cavity, pressure is exerted on the brainstem, resulting in a diminished level of consciousness, altered respiration, and, ultimately, cardiac arrest. Pressure on the cranial nerves, also located in this area, can lead to difficulty swallowing near the end of life. If swallowing difficulties occur early in the course of the disease, a formal swallowing evaluation should be performed and, if appropriate, enteral access devices, such as a percutaneous gastric tube, should be used. Late in the disease, such measures may not be indicated, particularly in lethargic or obtunded patients, given the discomfort that could be associated with these approaches and the diminished need for nutrition in these patients. Additionally, these measures add to neither comfort nor survival, making them of little value in the management of terminally ill patients. Alternate routes of medication administration other than enteral may be necessary to provide symptomatic relief, manage pain, and control seizures.

Conclusions

Optimal management of patients with brain metastasis involves, not only the treatment of the malignancy, but also the various deficits that are the physical manifestations of the disease. Patients should be the offered opportunity to participate in clinical trials whenever available, given the poor prognosis with most standard therapies and the potential for benefit from novel agents. Advances in therapy for primary malignancies will likely increase the overall survival of patients but with this comes the possibility of increasing the risk of brain metastasis. Thus, proper identification of symptoms, timely intervention, and, when appropriate, the institution of palliative care and hospice support should be part of the overall plan of management of these patients. The successful and compassionate management of symptoms can improve patient care at the end of life and make this process a tolerable and humane one for the patient and the family.

Acknowledgements

The authors thank David Galloway, Department of Scientific Publication, University of Texas M. D. Anderson Cancer Center.

References

1 Epstein, B. E., Scott, C. B., Sause, W. T. *et al.* (1993). Improved survival duration in patients with unresected solitary brain metastasis using accelerated hyperfractionated radiation therapy at total doses of 54.4 gray and greater. Results of Radiation Therapy Oncology Group 85–28. *Cancer* **71**, 1362–7.

2 Noordijk, E. M., Vecht, C. J., Haaxma-Reiche, H. *et al.* (1994). The choice of treatment of single brain metastasis should be based on extracranial tumor activity and age. *Int J Radiat Oncol Biol Phys* **29**, 711–17.

3 Patchell, R. A., Tibbs, P. A., Walsh, J. W. *et al.* (1990). A randomized trial of surgery in the treatment of single metastases to the brain. *N Engl J Med* **322**, 494–500.

4 Weinberg, J. S., Lang, F. F., and Sawaya, R. (2001). Surgical management of brain metastases. *Curr Oncol Rep* **3**, 476–83.

5 Shirato, H., Takamura, A., Tomita, M. *et al.* (1997). Stereotactic irradiation without whole-brain irradiation for single brain metastasis. *Int J Radiat Oncol Biol Phys* **37**, 385–91.

6 Auchter, R.M., Lamond, J.P., Alexander, E. *et al.* (1996). A multiinstitutional outcome and prognostic factor analysis of radiosurgery for resectable single brain metastasis. *Int J Radiat Oncol Biol Phys* **35**, 27–35.

7 Flickinger, J. C. (2001). Radiotherapy and radiosurgical management of brain metastases. *Curr Oncol Rep* **3**, 484–9.

8 Wen, P. Y. and Loeffler, J. S. (2000). Brain metastases. *Curr Treat Options Oncol* **1**, 447–58.

9 Kondziolka, D., Patel, A., Lunsford, L.D., Kassam, A., Flickinger, J.C. (1999). Stereotactic radiosurgery plus whole brain radiotherapy versus radiotherapy alone for patients with multiple brain metastases. *Int J Radiat Oncol Biol Phys* **45**, 427–34.

10 Bindal, R. K., Sawaya, R., Leavens, M. E. *et al.* (1993). Surgical treatment of multiple brain metastases. *J Neurosurg* **79**, 210–6.

11 Shaw, E., Scott, C., Souhami, L. *et al.* (2000). Single dose radiosurgical treatment of recurrent previously irradiated primary brain tumors and brain metastases: final report of RTOG protocol 90–05. *Int J Radiat Oncol Biol Phys* **47**, 291–8.

12 Postmus, P. E., Haaxma-Reiche, H., Smit, E. F. *et al.* (2000). Treatment of brain metastases of small-cell lung cancer: comparing teniposide and teniposide with whole-brain radiotherapy—a phase iii study of the European Organization for the Research and Treatment of Cancer Lung Cancer Cooperative Group. *J Clin Oncol* **18**, 3400–8.

13 Twelves, C.J., Souhami, R.L., Harper, P.G. *et al.* (1990). The response of cerebral metastases in small cell lung cancer to systemic chemotherapy. *Br J Cancer* **61**, 147–50.

14 Bernardo, G., Cuzzoni, Q., Strada, M.R. *et al.* (2002). First-line chemotherapy with vinorelbine, gemcitabine, and carboplatin in the treatment of brain metastases from non-small-cell lung cancer: a phase II study. *Cancer Invest* **20**, 293–302.

15 Antonadou, D., Paraskevaidis, M., Sarris, G. *et al.* (2002). Phase II randomized trial of temozolomide and concurrent radiotherapy in patients with brain metastases. *J Clin Oncol* **20**, 3644–50.

16 Hwu, W. J., Krown, S. E., Panageas, K. S. *et al.* (2002). Temozolomide plus thalidomide in patients with advanced melanoma: results of a dose-finding trial. *J Clin Oncol* **20**, 2610–5.

17 Gaspar, L., Scott, C., Rotman, M. *et al.* (1997). Recursive partitioning analysis (RPA) of prognostic factors in three Radiation Therapy Oncology Group (RTOG) brain metastases trials. *Intl J Rad Oncol Biol Physics* **37**, 745–51.

18 Christiaans, M.H., Kelder, J.C., Arnoldus, E.P., Tijssen, C.C. (2002). Prediction of intracranial metastases in cancer patients with headache. *Cancer* **94**, 2063–8.

Chapter 3

The prevention and treatment of seizures in intra-cranial malignancy

David Oliver

Summary

The prevention and correct treatment of seizures for patients with intra-cranial malignancy is an essential part of palliative care: seizures are a source of important concern for both the patient and their family and close carers. Prophylactic treatment of all patients with cerebral malignancy has not been shown to be necessary and great care should be taken with the prescription of anticonvulsants, as there are risks of interactions and adverse effects. Careful use of anticonvulsants should allow seizures to be controlled, and the fears of patient and family to be reduced.

Patients, their families and other carers should know how to carry out the initial treatment of a seizure. Clinicians should be prepared to act quickly to minimize the risk of status epilepticus, which has an appreciable morbidity and mortality, as well as being very distressing to witness.

The care of these patients requires effective multidisciplinary team work to ensure that the best possible control of seizures is achieved. This reduces the risk that families and carers will be left with frightening memories and complex problems in their bereavement.

Editor's note: In this chapter patient and family will be used to include unrelated but close carers and friends as well. Before discussing confidential medical details with family it is important that patients are happy to give permission.

Sources of evidence

The majority of studies concerned with the use of anticonvulsants are retrospective reviews. There has been one major review of the papers available from the Quality Standards Committee of the American Academy of Neurology,[1] which produced a practice parameter for the use of anticonvulsant prophylaxis.

Incidence

The reported incidence of seizures in cerebral tumours varies in the studies from 15 to 40%.[2] It has been estimated that 20–40% of patients present with a seizure, and a further 20–45% will ultimately develop seizures during the progression of the disease.[3] These figures demonstrate that many patients will experience a seizure during their illness—risking the physical and psychological health of the patient and distressing the family.

Assessment

A careful history is essential to make the diagnosis of seizures. It is important to exclude, and then treat, any potentially correctable causes of loss of consciousness that could be confused with a seizure. In particular:

- metabolic encephalopathies
- hyperglycaemia
- hypoglycaemia
- hyponatraemia
- hypomagnesaemia
- hypoxia.

Other possible causes include high doses of opioids or phenothiazines, cerebral infarction, or haemorrhage/transient ischaemic attack, alcohol abuse, or withdrawal and vaso-vagal attacks.

A full careful history, including details from someone who has observed a seizure, in conjunction with a physical examination and appropriate investigations, should exclude these causes. It is important to consider *all* the possible causes of a seizure, as they may occur concurrently in a patient with a known cerebral tumour.

Neuro-imaging, such as CT or MRI, will confirm the diagnosis of a cerebral tumour, and guide further management.

Management

The management of a seizure will depend upon whether this is a first episode or a recurrence of an earlier problem. The overall plan will be similar, as there is a need to assess each individual, and consider medication and other treatment options. The main primary treatment for seizures will be the use of anticonvulsant medication. However, this cannot be considered in isolation from the overall management of the patient and family, by the whole multidisciplinary team. It is important to explain, in appropriate detail, the possible implications of seizures to the patient and their family, including cerebral damage, the adverse psychological effects on the family—particularly children—of observing a seizure, and of the chance of aspiration, respiratory obstruction, and death. The need to stop driving should be emphasized. The risks and benefits of medication need explanation.

Corticosteroids

The use of corticosteroids is usual in these patients; there is a need to continually monitor the dose and consider the benefits of treatment. This area of care is complex and a wider multidisciplinary discussion is necessary, involving all involved in the care, including the patient and family. If there is a sudden onset of a seizure, or an increase in seizure frequency, this may reflect an increase in intra-cranial pressure, which may benefit from an increase in the dose of corticosteroid and, on occasions, radiotherapy may be indicated.

Both these areas need careful consideration. The likely benefits are better control of symptoms, including seizures and headache, but the risks include continuing to live a life of progressive disability and poor quality. These areas of discussion are not easy but the routine use of increased corticosteroids, without consideration of these wider concerns, should be avoided. The involvement of the patient, if they are able to discuss these issues, and their family with the wider multidisciplinary team is essential. The decision should, however, be taken by the professional team and should not be left to the family—it is an unenviable decision for a family to take and they may be left with regrets and concerns in their bereavement, if they feel they took responsibility for their relative's treatment.

Radiotherapy and surgery

Anticonvulsants should be prescribed prophylactically if radiotherapy is to be used, because the increase in peri-tumour oedema may increase the risk of further seizures. Surgery may be an option for a small minority of people with a single cerebral tumour, particularly benign tumours.

Anticonvulsant medication

The indications for the use of anticonvulsants in patients with cerebral tumours are far from clear. There are three main clinical situations to consider:

- patient presenting with a seizure;
- patient undergoing cranial irradiation or surgery;
- patient with a confirmed tumour but with no seizure.

These will be considered separately and the anticonvulsant drugs will then be described.

Patients presenting with a seizure

The benefits of using anticonvulsant medication are usually considered to outweigh the risks of medication. The increased risks of seizures, outlined above, are appreciable and therefore the side-effects of the medication are more acceptable. However, there may be significant interactions with other medication—in particular dexamethasone and chemotherapeutic drugs. The plasma levels of a number of anticonvulsants need to be monitored carefully in order to reduce the risks of underdosage—with ensuing seizures—or overdose—with potentially serious adverse effects.

Patients undergoing irradiation or surgery

There appears to be an increased risk of seizures during the period of irradiation and the use of prophylactic anticonvulsants should be considered during this time: they need to be continued for at least 2 weeks after the end of irradiation. The decision as to whether to continue with them after this time in patients who have never had a seizure will be considered below.

Patients undergoing surgery should receive anticonvulsants for a week before surgery, if possible, and continuing thereafter. The American Academy of Neurology Practice Parameter guidelines suggest that the dose should be reduced and stopped after a week, if the patient has not had a seizure, particularly in those patients who are medically stable and experiencing anticonvulsant-related side-effects.[1]

Patients who have never had a seizure

There have been many debates regarding the prophylactic use of anticonvulsant medication in patients with cerebral tumours.[1-3] Many neurological centres routinely use anticonvulsants, arguing that the prevention of seizures is important and that a large proportion of patients will develop them. However, the American Academy of Neurology review of the literature showed that there was no evidence that prophylactic medication was successful in reducing the number of seizures.[1] Moreover, there is increasing evidence that anticonvulsants, especially if the dose is not carefully monitored, may interact with corticosteroids and chemotherapeutic drugs leading to appreciable side-effects.[4] Many of the side-effects of over-dosage may be similar to those of tumour progression—such as ataxia, confusion, weakness—and this may confuse the future management of the patient. The Academy Practice Parameter recommends that 'anticonvulsants should not be used routinely in patients with newly diagnosed brain tumours'.[1]

The use of anticonvulsants

The choice of anticonvulsant frequently seems, in large part, to stem from the clinician's individual preference. There has been the tendency to use phenytoin but the slow build-up of plasma levels may be disadvantageous if control of seizures is required quickly. Sodium valproate and carbamazepine may be more effective and better tolerated.

Monotherapy is encouraged[5,6] and is usually effective for the majority of patients if plasma levels are monitored. It may be that the ineffectiveness of prophylaxis in seizure control shown in the literature was partly due to inadequate dosage regimens and thus plasma levels.[1] If seizures are not controlled by one anticonvulsant—usually carbamazepine or sodium valproate—at therapeutic plasma levels, a different drug should be substituted, slowly reducing the dose of the first drug as the new medication is introduced.[6]

If control is not obtained, vigabatrin may be substituted, or valproate and lamotrigine used in combination. Topiramate is another option. There is an increased risk of adverse effects with these anticonvulsants and the doses will need to be monitored very carefully.

It is essential to involve the patient (and their family, where appropriate) in the decisions regarding medication. They need to be aware firstly of the risks of treatment and, once medication has been started, on the need to continue on medication and to seek help if they are concerned that medication may be ineffective. At the end of life, if a patient is vomiting or has become so weak that oral medication can no longer be administered (see below), plasma levels may fall below the therapeutic range.

The occurrence of a seizure has a profound effect on the patient and their family. For many people, witnessing a seizure is a frightening event and the fear of further seizures can affect the relationships within a family. Seizures are still stigmatized, and patients and families may have some incorrect and unhelpful beliefs about them. Patients may feel embarrassed and ashamed if they have had a seizure in front of other people, particularly in a public place. The patient will also have to face not being allowed to drive, and for many this loss can be profound, and have consequences for their work and social lives. These concerns should be discussed openly and involve all those involved in the wider care of the patient and family.

Anticonvulsants

The main anticonvulsants in use for patients with cerebral tumours are given below.[6]

Phenytoin

Dose This should be 150–300 mg/day increasing to 600 mg/day, dose increases every 7–10 days. Usual dose 200–500 mg/day.

The bioavailability can vary from preparation to preparation and it is advisable to use the same formulation consistently. It may take a week to reach a measurable plasma level and several weeks to reach a therapeutic level. The medication should be taken with or after food.

Side-effects These can be varied and may be severe, including reduced appetite, headache, dizziness, gastro-intestinal upset, acne, hirsuitism, and gum hyperplasia. If the levels become toxic, there may be cerebellar, vestibular, and ocular disturbance leading to nystagmus, diplopia, slurred speech, and confusion. These symptoms may mimic the effects of the cerebral tumour and the monitoring of blood levels is essential.

Precautions Patients with liver dysfunction should be treated with care and in uraemia, protein-binding may be reduced, leading to toxicity.

Interactions There may be interactions with dextropropoxyphene and isoniazid. Anti-depressants can interact and lead to increased levels of phenytoin. Corticosteroids can lead to a higher or lower level of phenytoin and the efficacy of the steroids can be reduced; the bioavailability of dexamethasone can be reduced by 20% when phenytoin is started.

Sodium valproate

Dose The initial starting dose is usually 300 mg twice daily and the dose can be increased by 300 mg/day every three days to a therapeutic dose varying between 1 and 2 g/day. Blood levels should be monitored.

Side-effects It is generally well-tolerated, though gastro-intestinal side-effects, such as nausea and vomiting, may occur.

Precautions Care should be taken for patients with severe hepatic dysfunction.

Interactions Aspirin may increase plasma levels of valproate; there is a possible interaction with napoxen but the clinical relevance of this is uncertain.

Carbamazepine

Dose The initial dose is 100–200 mg/day and the dose should be increased slowly every 2 weeks to a maintenance dose of 800–1200 mg/day, with a maximum dose of 2 g/day. The total dose should be taken in two or four divided doses—with two doses the compliance may be increased but there may be a variation in the blood level over the 24-h period.

Side-effects These include dizziness, drowsiness, and ataxia, and are less common at lower dosages. If the plasma level is excessive, patients will become drowsy and suffer cerebellar and oculomotor dysfunction, leading to ataxia, diplopia, and nystagmus. Plasma levels should be monitored.

Precautions Care should be taken for patients with atrioventricular conduction problems and haematological disease.

Interactions Dextropropoxyphene and serotonin release inhibitor antidepressants can increase levels of carbamezepine. Lithium can cause neurotoxicity without an increase in drug levels. The metabolism of benzodiazepines may be enhanced as liver enzyme activity is enhanced. Corticosteroids are less effective as their clearance is increased, due to the induction of microsomal liver enzymes.

Vigabatrin

Dose This should be 1 g daily, increasing every week by 500 mg to a maximum of 3 g/day.

Side-effects Over 50% of patients develop side-effects, including drowsiness, fatigue, dizziness, nervousness, irritability, headache, nystagmus, ataxia, tremor, agitation, depression, and reduced memory. One-third develop an irreversible visual field defect.

Interactions There are many complex and severe interactions. These are unclear but care should be taken with any concurrent medication.

Lamotrigine

Dose The starting dose is 25 mg/day increasing by 25 mg every 2 days to a maximum of 500 mg/day.

If combined with other anticonvulsants, the initial dose is 50 mg/day increasing after 2 weeks to 50 mg twice daily to a usual maximum dose of 100 mg twice daily. Occasionally doses of up to 700 mg/day are necessary.

If combining lamotrigine with valproate, the initial dose is 25 mg every other day increasing to 25 mg daily after 2 weeks and then slowly increasing.

Side-effects These include skin rashes, diplopia, vision impairment, blood dyscrasias, and liver dysfunction.

Precautions Care is necessary for patients with hepatic or renal impairment—liver and renal function should be checked regularly.

Interactions Paracetamol may affect plasma levels.

Topiramate

Dose The starting dose is 25 mg/day, increasing by 25–50 mg every 1–2 weeks to a maximum of 200–400 mg/day in two divided doses.

Side-effects Ataxia, confusion, and dizziness may be seen.

Interactions Care should be taken with any concurrent medication. There may be an increase in toxicity without an increase in anti-epileptic activity; the interactions are very variable and unpredictable.[6] Phenytoin and carbamazepine appear to decrease the plasma level of topiramate.[6]

Status epilepticus

Status epilepticus can be defined as any epileptic seizure lasting longer than 30 min without recovery of consciousness—the fits may be generalized or partial in nature[7] The seizures that may occur are:

- tonic–clonic;
- epilepsia partialis continua (EPC), originating in the cerebral cortex and leading to clonic jerking of distal muscle groups, which may continue for weeks;
- complex non-convulsive status epilepticus—presenting as a confusional state without any obvious seizures.[7]

In status there is increasing frequency of seizures until they merge into continuous motor activity and there can be two phases:

The compensatory phase. There is increasing cerebral blood flow and metabolism to compensate and protect the brain. After 30 min, lactate levels may rise, cardiac rate and force of contraction increase, and there is hypertension and hyperglycaemia. Vomiting and hyperpyrexia may occur as a result of activation of the autonomic system.

The decompensatory phase. The compensatory mechanisms start to fail and cerebral blood flow and metabolism are reduced as a result of hypotension, and cerebral damage may occur, i.e. hypoxia occurs and cerebral oedema develops and cerebral damage may occur. Metabolic disturbances, including acidosis, hypoglycaemia, hypokalaemia, and hyponatraemia, can develop. Repeated convulsions may lead to rhabdomyolysis and this together with hyperuricaemia and acute tubular necrosis will cause renal failure.[7]

Status epilepticus has an appreciable mortality of up to 10%, although this is usually due to the effects of the underlying condition. Mortality is increased if treatment is delayed.

For the patient receiving palliative care, it may not be appropriate to manage the patient within intensive therapy facilities; but care can be provided within the hospital ward, hospice, or home setting. Benzodiazepines are the initial treatment—initially this may be by the rectal route (Stesolid enema 10–20 mg) and, if the seizures are not controlled, intravenous benzodiazepines, as emulsion 'Diazemuls' should be used:

- diazepam 10–20 mg at the rate of 5 mg/min;
- lorazepam 4 mg by slow injection;
- clonazepam 1 mg by slow injection.

Once the seizure has been controlled, maintenance treatment can be continued using midazolam—the usual dose is 10 mg as an initial injection subcutaneously followed by a continuous subcutaneous infusion using a syringe driver at a dose of 50–200 mg over 24 h.

There are concerns that there may be a 'ceiling' effect with benzodiazepines, as the GABA inhibitory system is maximally induced, so that increase in dosage may not have any improved effect;[8] other medication may then be necessary. It is also considered advisable to stop any phenothiazines, as these drugs may lower the epileptic threshold.

If the seizures are not controlled by benzodiazepines, phenobarbitone[9] should be considered as 200 mg by deep intramuscular injection. If this does not control the seizure, the dose can be increased by 50–100%.

The initial injection should be followed by a continuous subcutaneous infusion of phenobarbitone 600–2400 mg over 24 h.

If seizures continue, propofol has been suggested.[10] This is an anaesthetic agent and can give rapid sedation, although it can cause severe respiratory depression and the patient must be closely monitored. If the patient is at home, it may be necessary to consider transfer to an acute hospital, so that respiratory support is available.

Supporting the family is important during and after the episode. A loved one having continuous seizures is frightening to observers, who may also feel powerless. Advice on initial treatment—advice on the need to maintain the airway, by careful positioning of the patient during the seizure and the administration of rectal diazepam, is helpful, as this increases the sense of control of the situation.

Following an episode of status epilepticus it is essential to reassess the anticonvulsant therapy—starting regular medication if the patient has not received any before, or measuring the plasma levels and adjusting the dose of the existing medication, or changing or adding a further anticonvulsant.

Seizure management in the unconscious patient

As a patient with a cerebral tumour deteriorates, there may be increasing weakness and clouding of consciousness. Swallowing of medication may become increasingly difficult and continuation of oral anticonvulsants becomes impossible. Phenytoin and sodium valproate have long half-lives—22 and 20 h, respectively[6]—and a therapeutic level may be maintained. However, it is important to ensure control of seizures and other routes of administration should be considered:

- Initially medication may be given once to ensure seizure control:
  - rectal diazepam 10 mg;
  - subcutaneous midazolam 10 mg.
- After this initial dose, the anticonvulsant should be continued as:
  - diazepam as suppository 10–20 mg twice daily/ every 4 h;
  - midazolam 30–200 mg over 24 h as a continuous subcutaneous infusion by syringe driver;
- phenobarbitone 200–600 mg over 24 h by continuous subcutaneous infusion—this should usually be given alone, but can be mixed with diamorphine and hyoscine hydrobromide.[11]

The continuation of corticosteroids in the unconscious patient is a matter of debate. When the patient is unable to take the oral medication, steroids are not usually continued parenterally.[10] If there is felt to be an increased risk of seizure, headache, or distress—for instance, if there has been a recent episode of status epilepticus—dexamethasone may be continued, as an intra-muscular injection or a continuous subcutaneous infusion, at a low dose, to continue to help control raised intra-cranial pressure. However, this may also prolong the dying phase and these decisions need careful consideration by the multidisciplinary team caring for the patient.

Explanation and support of the family and close carers is essential so that they understand the rationale for continuing anticonvulsant medication, as they may feel that the patient is being over-sedated. However, they will usually appreciate the need to prevent further seizures.

As the patient deteriorates, the intra-cranial pressure may rise because they are no longer able to take corticosteroids or intra-cranial haemorrhage and the management would follow that for status epilepticus:

- rectal diazepam;

- intravenous diazepam (there are formulations available for IV use);

- subcutaneous midazolam—as a single injection followed by a subcutaneous infusion using a syring driver;

- phenobarbitone—as an initial injection intramuscularly and followed by a continuous subcutaneous infusion using a syringe driver.

The care of a person with intra-cranial malignancy requires a multidisciplinary approach and a careful assessment and use of medication, so that the most appropriate treatment is given.

References

1 Glantz, M. J., Cole, B. F., Forsyth, P. A. *et al.* (2000). Practice parameter: anticonvulsant prophylaxis in patients with newly diagnosed brain tumours. Report of the Quality Standards Subcommittee of the American Academy of Neurology. *Neurology* **54**, 1886–93.

2 Cohen, N., Strauss, G., Lew, R. *et al.* (1988). Should prophylactic anticonvulsants be administered to patients with newly-diagnosed cerebral metastases? A retrospective analysis. *J Clin Oncol* **6**, 1621–24.

3 Agbi, C. B. and Bernstein, M. (1993). Seizure prophylaxis for brain tumour patients: a brief review and guide for family physicians. *Can Fam Physician* **39**, 1153–64.

4 Gattis, W. A. and May, D. B. (1996). Possible interaction involving phenytoin, dexamethasone and antineoplastic agents: a case report and review. *Ann Pharmacother* **30**, 520–5.

5 Caracini, A. and Martini, C. (1998). Neurological problems. In *Oxford textbook of palliative medicine* (2nd edn) (ed. D. Doyle, G. W. C. Hanks, and N. MacDonald N), pp.737–8. Oxford University Press, Oxford.

6 Sweetman, S. (ed.) (2002). *Martindale: the complete drug reference* (33rd edn), pp.338–71.London, Pharmaceutical Press.

7 Hardy, J. R. and Martin, D. (2004). Neurological emergencies. In *Palliative care in Neurology* (ed. R. Voltz, J. L. Bernat, G. D. Borasio *et al.*). Oxford, Oxford University Press. In press.

8 Edwards, A. and Gerrard, G. (1998). The management of cerebral metastases *Eur J Pall Care* **5**, 7–11.

9 Stirling, L. C., Kurowska, A., and Tookman, A. (1999). The use of phenobarbitone in the management of agitation and seizures at the end of life. *J Pain Symptom Manage* **17**, 363–8.

10 Kuisma, M. and Roine, R. O. (1995). Propofol in the prehospital treatment of convulsive status epilepticus *Epilepsia* **36**, 1241–3.

11 Twycross, R. and Lichter, I. (1998). The terminal phase. In *Oxford textbook of palliative medicine* (2nd edn) (ed. D. Doyle, G. W. C. Hanks, and N. MacDonald N), pp.998–9. Oxford, Oxford University Press.

Chapter 4

The palliative management of raised intra-cranial pressure

F. A. Malik, E. J. Hall, and P. Edmonds

Introduction

There is very little evidence available on the palliative management of raised intra-cranial pressure caused by primary or secondary brain tumours. Most of the evidence on which this chapter is based comes from small case series, uncontrolled studies, and expert opinion, although one randomized controlled trial is discussed.

This chapter is concerned with adult malignancy, although some reference has been made to important differences between adults and children.

Scope of the problem

Of all adult cancer patients, 15–25% develop brain metastases (based on post-mortem studies). The median survival of patients with brain metastases is 2 months without treatment, depending on primary tumour type.[1]

Primary brain tumours are less common; for example, glioblastomas have an annual incidence of 5–12 per 100 000. The median survival for grade III anaplastic astrocytomas is 2 years and for glioblastomas 1 year.[2]

The percentage of adult patients with intra-cranial neoplasms who develop raised intra-cranial pressure (ICP) is unknown: in the studies available, the prevalence of individual symptoms has been recorded, rather than the syndrome of raised intra-cranial pressure.

Central nervous system (CNS) tumours account for 20% of the malignancies of childhood: 50% of these children survive in the long term. Approximately 25% of the children presenting with CNS tumours have the clinical features of raised intra-cranial pressure.[3]

Definition

Under resting conditions in a recumbent patient, the normal cerebrospinal fluid (CSF) pressure is between 0 and 10 mmHg. Some expert authorities would define a pressure of 20 mmHg or greater as raised intra-cranial pressure, while others use 15 mmHg as the upper limit of normal.[4]

Pathophysiology

Raised intra-cranial pressure is directly related to cerebral oedema, which is defined as an increase in brain volume due to an increase in water and sodium content. Vasogenic oedema is the type typically associated with cerebral neoplasms.

Hydrocephalus causes increased brain fluid due to impaired CSF absorption and may occur due to meningeal carcinomatosis or mechanical obstruction of the 4th ventricle by a posterior fossa tumour.

The mechanisms of vasogenic brain oedema are complex and are thought to arise from damage to the blood–brain barrier (BBB). There are many putative mechanisms and the relative contribution of these are not clearly known. As tumours enlarge they produce angiogenic factors that promote new capillary growth. Capillaries supplying metastatic brain tumours are fenestrated, lack tight junctions, and have an irregular basement membrane.

The disruption to the BBB results in it having an increased permeability to water-soluble substances and to large molecules such as proteins. These substances are driven into normal areas of the brain (predominantly white matter) by the increasing hydrostatic pressure and the effects are exacerbated by the lack of lymphatic drainage in the brain. The mean serum protein concentration in tissues is high in areas adjacent to glioblastomas and lower in those adjacent to metastases. The tumour-related capillaries not only produce angiogenesis of vessels that lack a normal BBB but also promote the leakiness of capillaries in normal brain tissue.

Arachidonic acid (AA) and its metabolites may play an important role in the promotion of vasogenic oedema. AA selectively increases capillary permeability within a tumour. It is a constituent of membrane phospholipids in the central nervous system but can also be produced in certain pathological conditions. Other molecules that contribute to these changes include bradykinin, histamines, leukotriene, free radicals, and serotonin.[1]

When hydrocephalus is present, the intra-cranial pressure is usually elevated unless the development has been gradual in onset. Rapid occlusion of the subarachnoid space by tumour particularly close to the sagittal sinus may elevate intra-cranial pressure whilst only causing mild ventricular dilatation.

Traction on pain-sensitive intra-cranial structures (e.g. the cranial nerves and dura) causes the headache associated with raised intra-cranial pressure. Damage to the brain parenchyma itself does not give rise to pain.

Assessment

History

Raised intra-cranial pressure (ICP) classically presents as a triad of headache, vomiting, and drowsiness. Patients with impending cerebral herniation may present as a neurological emergency with a more florid clinical picture.

Headache

In one series of 360 patients, headache occurred in 49% patients with brain metastases. The headache classically associated with raised ICP is said to occur early in the morning. The exacerbation of headache by coughing, sneezing, and bending is less common and occured in only 17% of patients in the same series.[1]

Headaches secondary to neoplasms occur more frequently in patients with a past history of headache. Older patients with atrophic brains are less likely to suffer headache.

Vomiting

This typically occurs when the patient wakes in the morning and may be projectile. The patient may not be nauseated.

Seizures

The proportion of patients presenting with seizures who also have raised intra-cranial pressure is small.

Cognitive impairment

This occurred in 58% of patients with raised ICP in one case series.[1]

Other problems

Carcinomatous meningitis can present with symptoms of raised intra-cranial pressure. Cranial nerve palsies are another common presenting feature of meningeal metastases. Single tumours located in particular areas will give rise to specific syndromes in addition to the symptoms of raised intra-cranial pressure. For example, depersonalization and behavioural changes may be subtle manifestations of frontal tumours, which can be mistaken for clinical depression. Other symptoms may include tinnitus, neck stiffness, paraesthesia, and back pain.

Hydrocephalus is a rare complication and presents as ataxia and confusion. The patient may also have other associated symptoms and signs caused by the underlying malignancy.

Onset

A rapid onset of symptoms at presentation suggests intra-tumoural haemorrhage or imminent cerebral herniation, which occurs in the direction of least resistance: through the foramen magnum or via transtentorial apertures.

Headache and somnolence occurring 6–16 weeks after cranial irradiation should be interpreted with caution: these are the cardinal symptoms of post-radiation sub-acute encephalopathy.

Children

The pattern of presentation in children is complex and non-specific, and this can lead to a delay between the onset of symptoms and confirmation of the diagnosis. Headache associated with a brain neoplasm is more common in children than adults—this is probably because there is a higher incidence of posterior fossa tumours in childhood. Other diagnostic symptoms include irritability, ataxia, unsteadiness, and progressive drowsiness.[3]

Examination

A full medical examination with careful assessment of the patient's neurological status should be performed. It is particularly important to identify:

- reduced level of consciousness;
- disorientation;
- focal neurological abnormalities;
- any signs related to the underlying primary malignancy.

Papilloedema occurs in about 20% of patients and probably reflects that the patient has had increased intra-cranial pressure for more than a few days. In this context, it does not usually cause visual defects. Visual field defects related to the tumour site may occur in up to 7% of patients. Papilloedema is more prevalent in children with brain tumours.

Other associated signs include bradycardia, hypertension, reduced respiratory rate, the stigmata of dehydration (from vomiting), and aspiration pneumonia.

Cranial nerve palsies are a common presentation of meningeal malignancy. It is important to remember that a palsy of the sixth nerve may represent a false localizing sign caused by tumour-related raised intra-cranial pressure.

Investigations

Making the diagnosis

If a patient presents with symptoms of raised intra-cranial pressure, it is vital to exclude potentially curable infections of the central nervous system, as these may mimic multiple brain metastases.

MRI (magnetic resonance imaging) with gadolinium is thought to be superior to CT (computed tomography) scanning,[5] especially for posterior fossa tumours. CT is cheaper and more readily available in the UK. In clinical practice in the UK, CT scanning is the most commonly used modality. Since many tumours demonstrate enhancement with contrast media, the use of intravenous contrast with CT scanning is recommended. Tumours can appear hypo, hyper or iso dense or there may be features of mixed density.

Editor's note: Where available MRI would be the investigation of first choice.

Other investigations

If brain metastases are diagnosed and these are the first presentation of malignancy, investigations to determine the site of the primary should be undertaken. Routine biochemical and haematological profiles should be requested to exclude factors that may exacerbate the symptoms of raised intra-cranial pressure and seizures; for example, hyponatraemia and hypo or hypercalcaemia (see Chapters 1 and 2 for more details on this).

Monitoring treatment

After palliative radiotherapy, routine neuro-imaging is usually only performed if there is an acute, unexpected deterioration, which may be caused by, for example, haemorrhage, hydrocephalus, or rapid disease progression. Neither CT nor MRI assists in the differentiation between tumour recurrence and radio-necrosis. Very occasionally, a cystic collection can cause deterioration, and this may be imaged and then drained neurosurgically. In a patient with a ventriculoperitoneal shunt, neuro-imaging may assist in diagnosis of a blocked shunt.

CSF pressure monitoring

Intra-cranial pressure monitors are used in the intensive care setting and can provide useful prognostic information, as well as monitoring the response to treatment and the patients' overall condition. Outside this setting, this technique is inappropriate.

Pharmacological treatment

Disease modifying treatment is discussed in Chapters 1 and 2.

Steroids

Background and mechanism of action

Adrenal glucocorticoids were first used in the management of oedema secondary to brain tumours in the late 1950s, although earlier animal studies indicated the potential effectiveness of glucocorticoids in this situation.

The mechanism of action has not been completely elucidated but their use results in stabilization of the BBB leading to a reduction in brain oedema. Potentially beneficial actions include:

- a direct effect on endothelial function leading to normalisation of vascular permeability;
- reduction of the filtration of plasma-derived fluid across tumour capillaries;
- reduction of the transport of albumin across the extra-cellular space;
- inhibition of arachidonic acid from cell membranes resulting in reduced production of oedema-related polyunsaturated acids;
- possible vasoconstrictive action;
- a possible direct anti-tumour effect, as well as an effect on increasing local cerebral perfusion and increasing the rate of CSF resorption;
- possible reduction in CSF formation may have a positive effect on increased intra-cranial pressure.

Some histological types of tumour respond better than others to steroids (e.g. metastatic tumours may be more steroid-responsive than gliomas). This may be related to the presence of specific glucocorticoid receptors in tumour cells. Steroids are ineffective in non-vasogenic brain oedema.

Symptom improvement can be seen initially 4–5 h post-steroid administration. However, the maximum effect most commonly occurs in 3–7 days.

For the first 24 h after dexamethasone administration, clinical improvement occurs even after a modest reduction in CSF pressure. Of patients with brain metastases, 70–80% respond to steroids.[6]

It is commonly thought that steroid-responsiveness is correlated with response to radiotherapy, however there is little evidence to support this. A clinical response to steroids is more marked in patients with evidence of generalized brain dysfunction, such as headache, papilloedema, and lethargy, and less dramatic for those with focal neurological signs.

The most effective dose regimen, type of corticosteroid, and duration of treatment cannot be established from the available research evidence.

Choice of steroid

Use of dexamethasone There are no controlled trials comparing the efficacy of one glucocorticoid against another but the most commonly used steroid remains dexamethasone, largely due to historical trials and theoretical benefits. Dexamethasone is least likely to cause fluid retention as it has minimal mineralocorticoid effects. The risk of infection may be also be reduced due to lesser inhibition of leucocyte migration. In addition, some experts state that the risk of cognitive and behavioural impairment is reduced compared with other steroids. However, as a fluorinated glucocorticoid, there appears to be a higher incidence of steroid myopathy.[1]

A dose of 1 mg dexamethasone is equivalent to 7.5 mg prednisolone, which gives it an advantage, as the number of tablets a patient is required to take is an important factor in the choice of steroid.

Pharmacology

Dexamethasone is well absorbed from the gastro-intestinal tract and undergoes first-pass metabolism in the liver. Drugs that induce liver enzymes, such as phenytoin, can reduce the systemic availability and therefore the efficacy of dexamethasone.

All steroids are highly protein-bound and therefore hypoalbuminaemia theoretically increases their bioavailability and, consequently, their side-effects.

Dexamethasone can be given orally, intravenously, intramuscularly, or subcutaneously (the latter is an 'off label' route). The parenteral route is favoured if the patient is vomiting or dysphagic or if a rapid onset of action is required. Prednisolone can be given orally and methylprednisolone is the parenteral equivalent. A comparison of the pharmacological properties of commonly prescribed steroids is detailed in Table 4.1.[1,7]

Table 4.1 Comparison of steroids[1,7]

Drug	Relative potency (glucocorticoid)	Relative potency (mineralocorticoid)	Equivalent anti-inflammatory dose (mg)	Biological half-life (hours)
Hydrocortisone	1	1	20	8–12
Prednisolone	4	0.25	5	18–36
Methylprednisolone	5	+_	4	36–54
Dexamethasone	25	+_	0.8	36–54
Fludrocortisone	10	300	—	18–36

Dose and duration of treatment

The most widely studied drug is dexamethasone and the following discussion applies to it.

There is no consensus on the optimal starting or maintenance dose of dexamethasone. However, bolus doses of 40–100 mg intravenously have been used to attempt to reverse imminent cerebral herniation or symptomatic patients with signs of instability.

In the United Kingdom palliative setting, the most commonly used starting dose is 16 mg/day. However, a randomized controlled trial demonstrated that a starting dose of 4 mg/day of dexamethasone led to similar improvements in performance status after 7 days when compared with 8 and 16 mg/day. The sample population in this study comprised 96 patients with radiologically proven brain metastases and a Karnofsky performance scale less than 80. There was a lower incidence of side-effects in the group taking 4 mg/day, compared with the group taking 16 mg/day.[8] Historical studies have led to the administration of dexamethasone in four divided doses per day, however the long biological half-life means that it can be logically given in a once or twice daily dose.

Anecdotal evidence supports the administration of steroids as early in the day as possible, to reduce potential sleep problems. The patient should be treated with the smallest effective dose for the shortest time possible to minimize side-effects. If steroids have been ineffective at controlling the symptoms of raised intra-cranial pressure within 5–7 days, they should be stopped.

Dose reduction

The timing of dose reduction will depend on whether there is surgical or oncological intervention as well. Radiotherapy can temporarily worsen oedema but there is no consensus on when to begin reducing steroids. One expert review suggests tapering should commence during the second week of radiotherapy. This paper proposes a schedule of dexamethasone at 16 mg/day for 4 days followed by 8 mg for 4 days, then a maintenance dose of 4 mg/day until radiotherapy is completed.[9]

Specialist oncological interventions are not appropriate for all patients— they may be too unwell, for example. In these patients dexamethasone should be reduced to the lowest effective dose as soon as possible. For example, a patient taking 16 mg of dexamethasone/day would be advised to reduce this by 2–4 mg every 5 days. There are, however, very wide variations in clinical practice and tapering is sometimes undertaken over a much shorter period.

Some clinicians make large initial reductions; for example, from 16 to 12 to 8 mg over a few days, then slow the rate of reduction to minimize the theoretical risk of adrenocortical suppression, which may occur at lower doses if there is a prolonged tapering period.

If a patient develops recurrent symptoms of raised intra-cranial pressure or evidence of steroid-withdrawal syndrome, the dose can be temporarily increased to the previous dose increment for 4–8 days before reducing again.[1]

Some clinicians would consider an increase up to 16 mg again for a trial period if symptoms recur, and consider staying at this dose if repeated attempts at tapering are unsuccessful. Indeed, it has been suggested that patients who have been on steroids for a number of months, and in whom tapering is difficult, the reduction schedule should be slower (e.g. 1–2 mg/week) to the lowest effective dose. There is no evidence to support any of these practices and the development of potentially severe side-effects with prolonged use must be balanced against symptomatic benefit.

All patients taking steroids should be issued with a blue steroid card (UK) and urged to show it to other health professionals involved in their care to make them aware of their steroid use.

Steroid withdrawal syndrome

There are a number of clinical problems that may be associated with reducing the dose of steroid or withdrawal of the drug.

Adrenal insufficiency This may develop when steroids are reduced too quickly, stopped suddenly, or if the patient experiences an intercurrent stressor, such as infection or surgery. At its most serious, this syndrome can present as an 'Addisonian crisis' with the patient presenting with sudden collapse and hypotension. Alternatively the presentation can be more insidious and mimic the symptoms and signs of the underlying brain tumour, such as headache, nausea, papilloedema, postural hypotension, and low-grade fever. Adrenocortical suppression from exogenous steroid use is more likely to occur after 10–14 days use.

Steroid pseudo-rheumatism This is the most common syndrome of steroid withdrawal and manifests as myalgia and/or arthralgia.

Pneumocystis carnii pneumonia This is a rare complication associated with steroid tapering: the exact mechanism is unknown.

Precautions when taking steroids Patients should be warned not to stop taking their steroids suddenly and that the dose may need to be temporarily increased if the patient suffers from inter-current infection, surgery, or other stressors.

Steroid side-effects

There is debate regarding whether the incidence of side-effects increases with duration and/or dose. In a recent study of dexamethasone use in 138 primary and secondary brain tumours, patients who complained of side-effects had been taking steroids for one week or more.[10] However, another retrospective study of 59 patients with either brain tumours or spinal cord compression showed that 76% of patients taking corticosteroids developed toxicity after three or more weeks of use.[11] A third of this sub-group developed their first toxic event in the first 3 weeks of therapy. The side-effects of steroids are shown in Table 4.2.

The figures for incidence of side-effects are taken from case series and retrospective studies with methodological flaws; for example, heterogeneous patient populations, varying doses of steroid, and multiple indications for steroid use.

Although some side-effects are potentially serious, they are of limited clinical relevance for patients with poor prognoses. For example, concerns about the development of osteoporosis or cataracts should not preclude their use in patients with a short life-expectancy. Steroid myopathy is potentially the most disabling side-effect in this group of patients and may reduce quality of life.

Table 4.3 outlines the frequency of steroid side-effects. The dosage and duration of steroid use varied in the three studies identified. Steroids were given for many indications, including neuro-oncological symptoms. In addition, definitions of side-effects varied and methods of identifying side-effects, e.g. hyperglycaemia, were not uniform across the studies. In children, growth retardation, altered body habitus, insatiable appetite, behaviour problems, and weight gain are important side-effects to monitor.

Management of side-effects

To minimize side-effects, the lowest effective dose should be used. One proposed schedule uses pulses of 8–16 mg for 5–7 days to limit side-effects;[7] this is common practice in children.

Oropharyngeal candidiasis responds to oral hygiene and anti-fungal agents. It is usual to prescribe a proton pump inhibitor to minimize gastro-intestinal side-effects, although there is no evidence to support this. It remains controversial whether steroids have ulcerogenic properties when given alone, but when given concomitantly with non-steroidal anti-inflammatory drugs, the risk of peptic ulceration is dramatically increased.[7]

Table 4.2 Steroid side-effects

Gastro-intestinal	Dyspepsia Peptic and oesophageal ulceration ($\uparrow$ if on anti-inflammatory drugs) Bowel perforation Abdominal distension Acute pancreatitis Nausea (very rare)
Musculoskeletal	Proximal myopathy Osteoporosis Avascular necrosis of bones Tendon rupture (Achilles especially)
Dermatological	Impaired wound healing Skin atrophy Bruising Striae Telengectasiae Acne
Endocrine	Adrenal suppression Menstrual irregularities Cushing's syndrome Hirsuitism Altered fat distribution (buffalo hump, moon face, weight gain)
Immunosuppression	Vulnerability to: candidiasis, pneumocystis carinii, chicken pox, tuberculosis
Neuropsychiatric	Euphoria Psychological dependence Depression Insomnia Psychosis Aggravation of pre-existing epilepsy
Blood	Leucocytosis Thrombo-embolism (rare)
Electrolyte/fluid balance	Sodium and water retention Hypertension Hypokalaemia
Ophthalmological	Glaucoma, papilloedema, cataracts, corneal and scleral thinning
Miscellaneous	Anaphylaxis (rare) Perineal tingling (after injection only) Malaise Hiccups

Table 4.3 Frequency of steroid side-effects

Side-effect	Study 1, $n = 138$[10]	Study 2, $n = 59$[11]	Study 3, $n = 109$[12]
Hyperglycaemia	56	11	4
Thrombo-embolism	4	N/k	N/k
Candidiasis	7	14	40
Pneumonia	1	N/k	N/k
Gastritis/Dyspepsia	4	3	7
Gastro-intestinal bleeding	0	4	N/k
Sigmoid perforation	N/k	1	N/k
Psychiatric	10	2	9
Peripheral oedema	8	5	20
Cushing's Syndrome	8	N/k	N/k
Myopathy	6	11	2
Skin changes	1	2	7

N/k = not known

To reduce insomnia and agitation, steroids should be given as early as possible in the day and a once or twice daily regimen used. Other practices to promote sleep at night ('sleep hygiene measures') should be adopted.

Steroid-induced psychosis, although rare, represents a psychiatric emergency requiring anti-psychotic drugs and cessation of the steroid as soon as possible.

Anecdotally prednisolone is associated with a lower risk of myopathy and a switch to this drug from dexamethasone may relieve symptoms if stopping the drug is not possible. In animal models, B vitamins and anabolic steroids have shown some benefit but this has not been translated into human studies. Graded exercise may help attenuate this problem.

There is no evidence to support the use of diuretics to reduce steroid-induced oedema; a time-limited trial of diuretics may be indicated in patients with severe oedema, but the patient must be monitored closely because of the risk of inducing intra-vascular volume depletion.

The dose of steroids in children There have been few attempts to study the optimum dose of steroids for children with central nervous system tumours. This is borne out by the lack of consensus in dose and duration of courses of steroid treatments. However, the initial response to steroids can sometimes be dramatic.

An audit of 62 paediatric patients receiving 130 courses of steroids revealed that 'short, sharp bursts' of dexamethasone 10 mg/m^2/day for 3–5 days may be useful for the control of symptoms for periods up to 4 weeks.[3] The consensus from this audit was to use steroids to maximize quality of life. They are usually used as an adjunct to further definitive therapeutic interventions such as surgical resection and debulking in addition to radiotherapy, but may have some role in the treatment of progressive neurological symptoms secondary to underlying disease.[3]

Osmotherapy

Uncertainty remains about the mode of action of osmotic agents in the management of raised intra-cranial pressure and cerebral circulation. It is thought that the effects of osmotherapy are related to the development of an osmotic gradient between blood and brain resulting in the shift of water producing a decreased brain volume and a lowered intra-cranial pressure. However, osmotic gradients obtained with hypertonic parenteral fluids do not last, because solutes reach an equilibrium concentration in the brain after a few hours and have a rapid metabolism.

Normal brain tissue has the capacity to shrink but areas of oedematous brain that are associated with increased capillary permeability remain unaffected. There is a risk of rebound phenomena as the solute does enter affected tissue and may increase tissue water.

In view of the rapid metabolism of these drugs, the rationale for chronic use in palliative care is debatable; it is more appropriate to use osmotic agents as a short-term measure prior to a definitive intervention, such as surgery. The osmotherapeutic agents commonly used are mannitol or glycerol. Mannitol, if effective, works within minutes, with a sustained effect lasting up to a few hours. Repeated doses are suggested if there is clinical deterioration, but their use may result in rebound phenomena.

Glycerol can be given orally and has been used in the longer-term management of brain oedema. It can lead to a reverse osmotic effect. There is no data of good quality to support its prolonged use in brain oedema secondary to tumours in a palliative population.

Diuretics such as acetozolamide and furosemide may be effective in vasogenic oedema. This is because the reduction in CSF formation could facilitate fluid drainage away from oedematous regions into the ventricular system. Furosemide and acetazolamide may inhibit CSF formation by between 25 and 50%. Acetozolamide is a carbonic anhydrase inhibitor, which reduces the availability of hydrogen ions for exchange with sodium ions in choroid plexus cells.

There is little evidence to support the use of diuretics in a palliative care population of patients with primary or secondary brain tumours. There is some evidence to suggest that a combination of mannitol and a loop diuretic can sustain and enhance the effect of mannitol in decreasing the ICP, although other experts state that furosemide has no 'role in the chronic management of tumour-related oedema'.[13] Loop diuretics show minor usefulness in oedema secondary to hydrocephalus.

Anti-emetics

There is no available evidence to support the superiority of one anti-emetic over another but in practice, the choice of anti-emetic is limited by potential side-effect profiles. Phenothiazines and butyrophenones should be used with caution because of the theoretical reduction in seizure threshold.

Cyclizine is theoretically the most useful anti-emetic for nausea and vomiting associated with raised intra-cranial pressure because it is thought to work at the vomiting pattern generator (vomiting centre), a diffuse neuronal network related to the lateral reticular formation and the midline medulla.

Corticosteroids are believed to have anti-emetic properties, in addition to the anti-oedema effects seen in raised intra-cranial pressure.

Other drugs used in palliative care of raised ICP

While steroids undoubtedly reduce headache and vomiting caused by raised intra-cranial pressure, other analgesics and anti-emetics are used in the palliation of these symptoms.

As with other cancer pain syndromes, the World Health Organization guidelines based on an analgesic ladder should provide the basis of pain management. However, there is some concern about the use of opioids in raised intra-cranial pressure for two reasons: they may mask symptoms of progressive disease, and theoretically may worsen headache by vasodilatation and increasing intra-cranial pressure.

There is some evidence to suggest that non-steroidal anti-inflammatory drugs are more effective in headache due to raised ICP. One small case series in non-malignant intra-cranial hypertension suggested that indomethacin reduced CSF pressure alongside improvement in symptoms, but there was no quantitative data on pain relief.[14]

Butyrophenones, anticonvulsants, and anti-depressants have been used in non-malignant headache, but there are no studies of efficacy in malignant headache. Concern about the reduction of seizure threshold by butyrophenones and anti-depressants limit their potential use.

Acupuncture has been studied in non-malignant headache and found to be of benefit in a recent critical review[15] but further research is required to clarify efficacy and safety in patients with malignant headache.

Anticonvulsants for seizure reduction are discussed elsewhere in this book.

Non-pharmacological management

Shunts

Hydrocephalus may be caused by posterior fossa tumours or leptomeningeal metastases (most commonly from breast, lung, and lymphoma primaries). It is a rare complication in adults.

In one case series, the authors comment on the lack of availability of data on the use of ventriculo-peritoneal shunting as a palliative surgical procedure for this problem.[16] They report on two patients with non-small lung cancer and one with breast cancer who had ventriculo-peritoneal shunts placed for symptomatic hydrocephalus. All three patients had resolution of symptoms, including return of a normal gait and relief of headache. Only one patient had abnormal mentation, but this improved. However, two had other specialist oncological treatments as well.

The indications for shunt insertion in adults with cerebral malignancy remain uncertain. Adverse effects include infection, blockage, pulmonary hypertension (ventriculo-atrial shunts), and a potential risk of seeding of metastases into the peritoneal cavity.

Hyperventilation

Hyperventilation may be used as a non-pharmacological intervention in an attempt to rapidly decrease raised intra-cranial pressure in an intensive care setting in hospital, although this is rarely appropriate or feasible in patients requiring palliative care.

Hyperventilation decreases the partial pressure of carbon dioxide in undamaged areas of brain. Carbon dioxide causes vasodilatation and can contribute to an increase in cerebral blood volume and flow resulting in increased intra-cranial pressure. Hyperventilation causes a rapid lowering of ICP that can last for 15–20 min. Hyperventilation requires intubation of the patient and ventilation is required to decrease the partial pressure of CO_2 to 25–30 mmHg. Mechanical ventilation may result in an increase in ICP particularly in patients with brain lesions.

Palliative care issues

Palliative care requires a multi-professional approach and focuses on maintaining and improving quality of life, and therefore patients' priorities and goals are the key concerns. It is therefore essential to make sure that patients fully understand the treatment options available to them and that family are involved (as the patient allows) in helping to make choices. Symptom control and support of the patient and family is central at all stages of the disease trajectory. Optimal symptom control requires the use of the pharmacological and non-pharmacological approaches as outlined above.

Cognitive impairment can occur as part of the disease process and therefore thinking and planning ahead should be encouraged; for example the use of advanced directives, setting up an enduring power of attorney, making a will, and so on.

As it is so difficult to predict accurately the disease trajectory and prognosis, it is important to consider the risks and benefits of both further anticancer therapy and antibiotic use at each stage of the illness. For example, in a patient with a short prognosis who has an important social occasion, one might consider the use of steroids, antibiotics, or osmotherapy in an attempt to reach this goal.

It is important to offer information about potential developments during the illness, such as warning patients and carers of possible personality changes and challenging behaviour. Community palliative care teams have the expertise to offer support in the patient's home and can liase with the other professionals involved in the care of the patient. There should be an agreed plan among professionals, patients, and carers about steroid dosage changes in relation to the patient's condition.

For those patients presenting with clinical evidence of raised ICP, but who are also clearly dying, the use of steroids may be inappropriate. Such treatment decisions require careful consultation with the patient (if possible), and carers and healthcare professionals who have previously been involved with the patient's care.

Management of the terminal phase

In the last few days of a patient's life, admission to an in-patient unit may be necessary if symptoms cannot be controlled in the home or the patient or carer is distressed. More information on this can be found in Chapter 9.

Unnecessary oral medication should be discontinued. There is considerable variation in practice regarding the reduction or cessation of steroids in the last few days of life. Table 4.4 outlines the results of a survey of dexamethasone use

Table 4.4 Use of dexamethasone in the last days of life[17]

Time (days before death)	Dexamethasone dose (mg/day) mean (range)
14	7.9 (0–16)
7	7.2 (0–20)
2	5.2 (0–24)
1	2.9 (0–24)

in the last 14 days of life in primary brain tumour patients in eight hospices and one cancer centre.

Altogether 7 (11 %) patients did not receive dexamethasone in the last 14 days of life and in 15 patients (23%) dexamethasone was stopped when they could no longer swallow. In 16 patients (24%) dexamethasone was increased in order to reverse clinical deterioration or relieve the effects of raised intra-cranial pressure in the last 14 days of life.

Another retrospective review of corticosteroid use at the end of life investigated all deaths in a hospice over a 6-month period.[18] Steroid use at the end of life was found to be common. The main indications were to reduce raised intra-cranial pressure and promote well-being. Of patients prescribed steroids during their terminal admission, 61% received steroids on the day of their death. This study highlighted the need for regular review of corticosteroid prescribing.

Terminal care guidelines are currently being developed for children at home but should be considered for all patients. Access to emergency drugs, such as diamorphine, midazolam, and diazepam, should be available at any time. These drugs could be included in a crisis box for use in the home, if appropriate. Carers should be offered education about rectal and buccal routes of administration.

Sensitive discussions about the appropriate use of parenteral fluids should take into account benefits and burdens of these in the last few days of life. Parenteral fluids can increase intra-cranial pressure and therefore may worsen oedema-related headache.

Cerebral irritation may manifest as agitation, seizures, twitching, and can be treated with benzodiazepines. However, other potentially remediable causes of terminal restlessness should always be excluded; for example, uncontrolled pain or urinary retention. The most commonly used agents for cerebral irritation are midazolam or clonazepam, which have anticonvulsant as well as anxiolytic and sedative properties.

For patients previously on oral anticonvulsants, who can no longer swallow, suitable starting doses are 20–30 mg of midazolam or 2–4 mg of clonazepam/ 24 h subcutaneously. Phenothiazines and butyrophenones are used for the management of terminal restlessness but should be avoided if possible in patients who have had seizures. For severe uncontrolled agitation, other options include phenobarbitone (600–2400 mg/24 h subcutaneously) or propofol.

Psychological considerations

It can be very difficult to distinguish between radiotherapy or steroid-induced psychiatric symptoms and depressive symptoms. In addition the anatomical location of the tumour may result in neuro-psychiatric symptoms.

There is limited data on diagnosis of major depressive disorders in adult patients with brain tumours. One American study of 89 patients with primary brain tumours in neuro-oncology out-patient clinics suggested that 28% of patients fitted DSM-IV criteria for major depressive disorder.[19]

The incidence was higher in those with frontal lobe tumours and those with a family history of psychiatric disorder. Lesions in the temporal lobe and limbic systems may result in mania, panic attacks, amnesia, or hallucinations. Anxiety and depression are found more frequently in tumours of the left hemisphere.

Carers of patients with brain tumours may be more psychologically vulnerable, especially if the patient had personality changes, cognitive deficits, or challenging behaviour.

More discussion on these topics can be found in Chapters 5 and 6.

Other specialists who may help

Palliative care requires the skills of a multi-professional team. In addition to doctors and nurses other professionals who can help with caring for patients with the patient with raised intra-cranial pressure include:

- physiotherapists who can assist in maintaining mobility, balance, and managing respiratory symptoms, while occupational therapists can advise on specialist equipment and discharge planning;
- day-centre staff and volunteers offer respite for carers and constructive activities for patients;
- social workers, counsellors, and other psychological therapists can provide practical advice and emotional support to patients and carers.

Palliative-care services may also offer complementary therapies such as therapeutic massage, acupuncture, hypnotherapy, and aromatherapy, which may be very helpful for patients and families.

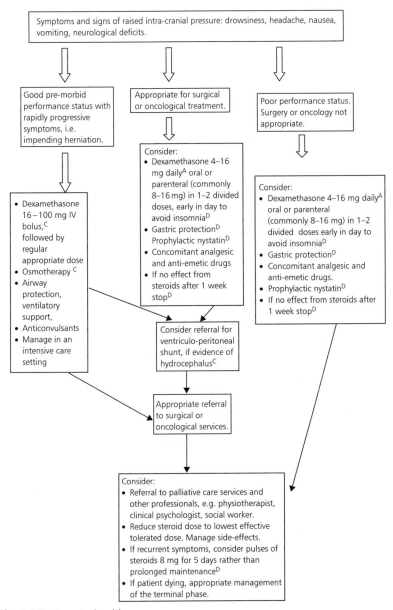

Fig. 4.1 Treatment algorithm.

NOTE: The letters in superscript refer to recommendations based on levels of evidence according to the US agency for health care policy.[20]

A = meta-analysis or at least one randomized controlled trial

B = Non-randomized studies or non-experimental descriptive study

C = Expert opinions/committees

D = Anecdotal

Liaison with other teams and services

The management of raised intra-cranial pressure involves neuro-oncologists, neurosurgeons, and radiologists working closely with palliative-care specialists and family physicians (GPs), so that the patients' goals of treatment are clearly understood and kept in mind when different therapeutic options are considered.

Close liaison with community teams must be maintained, as most patients will want to spend as much time at home as they can, living as normally as possible. The time will come when specialist oncological and neurosurgical interventions will no longer offer the best chance of effective palliation of this condition, and other palliative treatments become more important. The family physician will often want specialist palliative care or oncological advice about the best treatment options and access to this is key to good community care.

A treatment algorithm is shown in Fig. 4.1.

References

1 Posner, J. B. (1995). *Neurologic complications of cancer*, pp.3–10, 37–54, 59–66, and 77–96. FA Davis Publishing.

2 Rees, J. (2002). Glioma therapy. *Advances Clin Neuro Rehab* **2** (2), 11.

3 Glaser, A., Buxton, N., and Walker, D. (1987). Corticosteroids in the management of CNS tumours. *Arch Dis Childhood* **76**, 76–8.

4 Lundberg, N. (1960). Continuous recording of ventricular fluid pressure in neurosurgical practice. *Acta Psychiatr Neurol Scand* **36** (149), 1–193.

5 Hoskin, P. J. and Brada, M. (2001). Consensus report: radiotherapy for brain metastases: *Clinical Oncology* **13**, 91–4.

6 Weissman, D. E. (1988). Glucocorticoid treatment for brain metastases and epidural spinal cord compression. *J Clin Onc* **6** (3), 543–51.

7 Hardy J. (1998). Corticosteroids in palliative care. *Eur J Palliat Care* **5**, 46–50.

8 Vecht, C. J., Hovestadt, A., Verbiest, H. B. C. *et al.* (1994). Dose-effect relationship of dexamethasone on Karnofsky performance in metastatic brain tumours. *Neurology* **44**, 675–80.

9 Weissman, D. E., Janjan, N. A., Erickson, B. *et al.* (1991). Twice-daily tapering dexamethasone treatment during cranial radiation for newly diagnosed brain metastases. *J Neuro-Oncol* **11**, 235–9.

10 Hempen, C., Weiss, E,. and Hess, C. F. (2002). Dexamethasone treatment in patients with brain metastases and primary brain tumours: do the benefits outweigh the side-effects. *Supp Can Care* **10** (4), 322–8.

11 Weissman, D. E., Dufer, D., Vogel, V. *et al.* (1987). Corticosteroid toxicity in neuro-oncology patients. *J Neuro-Oncol* **5**, 125–8.

12 Hanks, J. G. W., Trueman, T., and Twycross, R. G. (1983). Corticosteroids in terminal cancer—a prospective analysis of current practice. *Postgraduate Medical Journal* **59**, 702–6.

13 DeAngelis, L. (1994). Management of brain metastases. *Cancer Investigation* **12** (2), 156–65.

14 Forderreuther, S. and Straube, A. (2000). Indomethacin reduces CSF pressure in intra-cranial hypertension. *Neurology* **55**, 1043–5.

15 Manias, P., Tagaris, G., and Karageorgiou, K. (2000). Acupuncture in headache: a critical review. *Clinical J Pain* **16**, 334–9.

16 Lokich, J., Levine, H., and Nasser, I. (1998). Malignancy-related hydrocephalus: clinical features and results of ventricular peritoneal shunt procedure in three patients. *Am J Clin Oncol* **21** (4), 366–8.

17 Wand, P. J. and Campbell, C. (2000). *Dexamethasone administration in the last 14 days of life in patients dying of primary brain tumours.* Poster, 1st Congress of Research Network of the European Association for Palliative Care, Berlin, December.

18 Gannon, C. and McNamara, P. (2002). A retrospective observation of corticosteroid use at the end of life in a hospice. *J Pain Symptom Manage* **24**, 328–34.

19 Wellisch, D. K., Kaleita, T. A., Freeman, D. *et al.* (2002). Predicting major depression in brain tumor patients. *Psycho-Oncol* **11**, 230–8.

20 US Agency for Health Care Policy and Research. (1993). *Acute pain management: operative or medical procedures and trauma* (Clinical Practice Guideline No. 1) (AHCPR Publication No. 92-0023), p. 107.

Chapter 5

Neuropsychological complications in patients with brain tumours

Anne E. Kayl and Christina A. Meyers

Introduction

Individuals diagnosed with primary or metastatic brain tumours face a difficult battle, and one that will likely be fought on several fronts. In addition to the physical effects of the disease and treatment-related discomfort, brain tumours often cause profound changes in cognitive function, personality, and psychological well-being.

As the disease progresses and treatment side-effects become more pronounced, family roles may change, patient productivity may decline, and self-esteem may suffer. To provide comprehensive care of patients with brain tumours, the modern practitioner must address the psychological, as well as the biological, implications of the disease. An appreciation of the cognitive deficits and behavioural changes that may occur with this diagnosis will aid intervention strategies, improve the quality of patient care, and ultimately improve the overall quality of life for brain tumour patients and their families.

Neurobehavioural changes due to brain tumours

For patients and their families, who are just coming to terms with the diagnosis of brain tumour, emotions such as disbelief, anger, confusion, and anxiety run high. Eventually, questions regarding the potential impact of the disease on cognitive function are raised. Unfortunately, predicting the nature and severity of cognitive impact is difficult, since the cognitive and behavioural profiles of brain tumour patients can vary tremendously, despite commonalities of tumour histology or location. Although not as well studied as primary tumour populations, in our experience, patients diagnosed with metastatic brain tumours frequently evidence impairment of cognitive and motor functioning, and these impairments often pre-date the initiation of treatment.

Tumour location

Dysfunction of specific brain regions may lead to predictable cognitive deficits. For instance, left-hemisphere tumours are commonly associated with language disorders that impair the patient's ability to communicate with others and comprehend spoken or written language, while tumours located in the right hemisphere are more likely to cause deficits of visual perception or visual scanning.

Disturbances of executive functions (manifested by impairments of cognitive flexibility, abstraction, motivation, planning and organizational skills, ability to benefit from experience, personality changes, etc.) are frequently associated with tumours of the frontal lobes. However, executive deficits are not limited to patients with frontal-lobe tumours. In some cases, non-frontal tumours disrupt afferent and efferent frontal-lobe connections, effectively disrupting modulatory frontal influences. The site of the brain tumour also has an impact on mood. Patients with tumours in ventromedial frontal or parietal association areas are more likely to experience anxiety, irritability, and fatigue, while emotional indifference is most often associated with dorsolateral frontal and somatosensory region lesions.

Tumour pathology

Because the brain has a remarkable ability to adapt, persons diagnosed with slowly developing tumours may have few detectable changes in brain function. In contrast, patients with very rapidly growing tumours may have widespread impairment due to mass effect on adjacent brain regions. Although early studies suggested that patients with more malignant tumours evidence more severe impairment of cognitive function,[1] we have found that statistically controlling for tumour size eliminates any differences in the cognitive profiles of patients with rapidly- vs. slowly-growing tumours.[2]

Neurobehavioural changes due to treatment

Cognitive dysfunction in brain tumour patients is often more generalized than expected for a focal lesion. In addition to tumour-related factors, there may be different adverse effects attributable to radiation, chemotherapy, immunotherapy, and adjunctive medications.

Adverse effects of radiation

The majority of patients diagnosed with malignant brain tumours will undergo radiotherapy at some point during their illness. As treatment progresses, many patients experience significant fatigue. Such fatigue may be reflected in slowed or more effortful thinking, in addition to an increased need for rest. Fortunately, the majority of patients will note improvement in their energy levels and stamina once radiotherapy is complete.

Brain irradiation may also be associated with delayed changes in brain tissue and cognitive deficits. The damage from radiation treatments is generally evident a year or more following treatment, and may be progressive and irreversible. The area of injury may present as an expanding mass of necrosis that is virtually indistinguishable from recurrent tumour, or as diffuse progressive white-matter disease (leukoencephalopathy). Older patients, young children, and individuals who receive concomitant high-dose chemotherapy, are at greatest risk for suffering from the adverse effects of radiation. Treatment-related changes may include gait disturbance, weakness, and tremor. In addition, cognitive declines in information-processing speed, executive functions, memory, and sustained attention are not uncommon.

Whole brain radiotherapy (WBRT) has been used in the management of metastatic brain lesions for many years and may be used as a primary therapy or after surgical resection or stereotactic radiosurgery. Cognitive disturbances and side-effect severity are generally related to such variables as total radiation dose and dosing interval. The acute and sub-acute effects (i.e. hair loss, headaches, vomiting, and lethargy) of WBRT can be troublesome and persistent. However, the late effects of WBRT can be more debilitating and can include radiation necrosis, brain atrophy, white-matter changes, and significant cognitive decline.

Adverse effects of chemotherapy

Cognitive and emotional changes reported during and after chemotherapy include memory loss, decreased information-processing speed, reduced attention, anxiety, depression, and fatigue. Most of the older literature suggests that neurotoxic side-effects of chemotherapy are acute and reversible, generally resolving within 48–72 h after treatment. The risk of severe delayed effects, such as leukoencephalopathy, is primarily seen following higher doses, intra-arterial or intra-ventricular administration, and concomitant radiation therapy. The neurobehavioural effects of most cancer therapy agents tend to be non-specific and diffuse, except for those that have a mechanism of action that is expected to affect focal brain regions or biologic response modifiers that are known to affect particular pro-inflammatory cytokines, neurotransmitters, and neuro-endocrine hormones.

Adverse effects of immunotherapy

Cytokines, such as interferon alpha (IFN-α) and interleukin-2 (IL-2), have been used in a number of therapeutic trials for primary brain tumours and leptomeningeal disease (LMD). These agents are known to have both acute and persistent neurotoxic side-effects. Acute toxicity is characterized by fever, headache, and myalgia, which generally resolves over several days. Sub-acute neurotoxicity, evident within a week of starting therapy, is characterized by inattention, slowed thinking, and lack of motivation. After several months of treatment, more than two-thirds of patients develop difficulty with memory, frontal-lobe executive functions (e.g. problem-solving, planning, sequencing), motor coordination, and mood,[3] and these neurotoxic side-effects are not always reversible following treatment cessation.[4] The route of administration is also an important consideration. Intra-ventricular administration of IFN-α has caused a reversible vegetative state in patients with LMD,[5] and intra-ventricularly administered IL-2 may produce a progressive dementia in otherwise 'cured' patients treated for LMD.[6]

Adverse effects of adjunctive medications

Steroids

Glucocorticoid treatment for mass effect and raised intra-cranial pressure is ubiquitous in brain tumour patients. However, steroids may also have adverse effects on mental and emotional functioning. The incidence of steroid-induced psychiatric syndromes ranges from 5.7% to 50%.[7] These side-effects include euphoria, mania, insomnia, restlessness, and increased motor activity. Increased levels of anxiety, depression, and memory problems are also common complaints among patients in our clinic.

Anticonvulsants

When the dosages of anticonvulsant drugs such as phenytoin (Dilantin) and carbamazapine (Tegretol) are carefully monitored, their cognitive effects are minimal. Use of phenobarbital, however, has been associated with greater adverse cognitive effects. Regardless of the specific medication used, too rapid introduction of the anticonvulsant, polypharmacy, or excessive concentrations may result in changes in arousal, attention, memory, and psychomotor functioning.[8] It should be noted, however, that the majority of children and adults who take these drugs experience few (if any) side-effects. In fact, at least one anti-epileptic drug appears to have favourable effects on psychological well-being.[9]

Specific medical and behavioural concerns

Delirium

Delirium is a common problem among patients with advanced cancer and presentation of the condition may vary tremendously across individuals.

Altered consciousness is the hallmark of delirium, but most patients also present with disturbances of attention, memory, and other cognitive functions. Delirium may present as a sudden decline in arousal and activity levels, but dramatic elevations of arousal are also possible. Among cancer patients, common causes of delirium include metabolic disturbances (i.e. hyponaetremia, hypercalcemia) and CNS infection. Increased intra-cranial pressure may also cause changes in arousal levels. Once the source of the problem is identified and treatment is initiated, symptoms of this disorder typically show rapid improvement.

Emotional changes

Various factors, including biological, environmental, and personality traits, contribute to behaviour problems in persons diagnosed with brain tumours. Behavioural disinhibition and impulsive tendencies are commonly associated with tumours of the orbitofrontal cortex, while damage to ventromedial frontal regions has been associated with lack of initiation and apathy. Depression and adjustment disorders are common diagnoses among cancer patients and may be managed with medication, psychotherapy, or a combination of treatments. Although increased irritability is a frequent complaint of patients seen by our service, frank aggression is relatively rare. In some cases, the patient is unaware of behaviour changes, but they can be quite distressing to family members. Fortunately, there are skills and strategies that are relatively easily employed and can reduce the frequency of inappropriate or maladaptive behaviours, as well as increase the frequency of adaptive responses.

Gaining control over the patient's environment can frequently reduce the incidence of problematic behaviours. For example, improvements in lighting, reduction of noise, and limiting the number of visitors in the patient's room, all reduce the likelihood of over-stimulation and agitation during hospital stays. In both in-patient and out-patient settings, family members are encouraged to ignore inappropriate behaviours and to reward adaptive responses. To encourage activity and social involvement, we ask caregivers to use direct, concrete requests (i.e. 'Please set the table' vs. 'Please help me get ready for dinner') for assistance. Family members are also taught to recognize signs of increasing irritability and learn when to redirect the patient's attention and when to simply back off and try again in a few minutes.

These are but a few of the strategies and techniques that may be useful for patients and their caregivers. Development of a treatment plan should be individualized and evolve from an understanding of the organic, environmental, and personality factors that contribute to the problematic behaviour.

Cognitive rehabilitation and compensatory techniques

It is almost certain that rehabilitation could reduce disease-related morbidity and improve the cognitive and emotional function of brain tumour patients, but programs for this group remain in the early stages of development. At this time there is little established knowledge about the major rehabilitation problem areas of brain tumour patients and no rehabilitation approaches to address the problems that have been specifically validated in this clinical population.

Pharmacological strategies

Neurobehavioural slowing is the hallmark of frontal-lobe dysfunction and treatment-related adverse effects in brain tumour patients. The syndrome of neurobehavioural slowing is generally due to involvement of the monamine pathways of the frontal–brainstem reticular system. In addition, catecholamines have an important role in the modulation of attention and working memory.

Stimulant (methylphenidate) treatment has proven useful in the treatment of concentration difficulties, psychomotor retardation, and fatigue frequently seen in brain tumour patients, and helped to elevate mood as well.[10] A conservative dose of 10 mg twice daily significantly improved cognitive function as assessed by objective tests, and doses in excess of 60 mg twice daily were well tolerated. Subjective improvements included improved gait, increased stamina and motivation to perform activities, and improved bladder control. There were no significant side-effects, and many patients taking steroids were able to decrease their dose. Long-term experience with this agent is lacking to determine if tolerance to therapeutic effects can develop.

Cognitive remediation

It is clear that patients with brain tumours may benefit from a variety of rehabilitation services including physical therapy, occupational therapy, and speech and language therapy. However, the types of problems facing this group are quite different from the challenges facing other patient groups. In a survey of 30 caregivers of brain tumour patients (unpublished data), we found that the most salient problems facing brain tumour patients were lack of energy, inability to perform usual activities around the home (i.e. paying bills, making repairs), social isolation, lack of sexual activity, generalized slowing of behaviour, and problems with reasoning, memory, and concentration.

The majority of the brain tumour patients seen in our clinic are experiencing cognitive difficulties. Feelings of confusion and frustration often accompany cognitive changes and can affect not only the patient, but also those close to him or her.

For many patients, whether they are newly diagnosed or already in treatment, a neuropsychological assessment can be helpful in delineating the individual patient's cognitive strengths and weaknesses, as well as validate the concerns of patients and their families. In some instances, the neuropsychological evaluation provides concrete evidence of impairment for the patient who is unable or unwilling to acknowledge that impact of the disease and/or their treatment on cognition.

Many of our patients reside out-of-state or at a distance from the facility that prohibits frequent visits for cognitive remediation. Although referrals to accredited rehabilitation facilities are provided when appropriate, some patients benefit from an intensive 'problem-solving' approach that can be completed in conjunction with scheduled clinic visits. With this type of supportive approach, emphasis is placed on providing the patient and the caregivers with simple, concrete strategies for managing cognitive deficits. For instance, memory impairments may be managed with a 'memory notebook' designed and organized for the individual patient.

We often advocate the use of large-print calendars in the home to improve patient orientation and enable them to remain more aware of daily schedules. Tape recorders can be used during patient–doctor meetings and reviewed at a later time to enhance patient recall, comprehension, and compliance with treatment recommendations. When possible, family members are enlisted as 'co-therapists' and instructed in techniques to be used at home.

More structured programs are available for patients who reside within easy commuting distance from the hospital. For these patients, cognitive rehabilitation begins with an assessment of simple visual and auditory attention skills. Difficulty in one of these areas will hamper the 'higher' mental functions. For instance, how can a patient learn, respond appropriately, and otherwise function to their potential if they are inaccurately perceiving incoming information? Once cognitive impairments are identified through a formal neuropsychological assessment, an individualized treatment plan is developed. The plan is developed over one or two sessions and considers the input of the patient, their family members or support system, and the neuropsychologist. In some cases, remedial work in visual and auditory attention is required. Once these foundation skills are maximized, we address the more complex functions such as memory, problem-solving skills and visuospatial abilities.

Many of the previously mentioned strategies and aids are useful in the in-patient setting, as well. For example, all patient rooms should be equipped with a large print, dry-erase calendar. Basic orientation information should be clearly posted (with timely updates), along with the names of those involved in their care. In a similar vein, healthcare professionals should never assume that the patient remembers their name or their role. Frequent re-introductions and 'talking through' medical procedures before drawing blood, or before relocating the patient for tests, can greatly alleviate patient anxiety and improve compliance rates. Providing written information on upcoming procedures or treatment plans is also helpful. For the patient with a visual neglect, simply orienting the bed so that people enter on the attended to side may relieve anxiety and make interactions more enjoyable. Although these points may seem to be 'common sense', they are often forgotten in the course of a busy day.

In our experience, families of brain tumour patients are burdened by the patients' cognitive and behavioural changes in addition to the typical psychological problems of coping with cancer in a family member. They may have particular difficulty dealing with neurologically caused personality changes, such as loss of initiative, quick mood changes, loss of control over emotions, and lack of insight into limitations. Support groups for brain tumour patients and their family members may be of great benefit. In our support group, one meeting a month is devoted to a topic discussion or lecture on an area of interest such as seizure medications. The other meeting each month is for open discussion and is more supportive in nature. Similar programmes are becoming available at other cancer centres, partly through the advocacy efforts of the National Brain Tumour Foundation.

The previous discussion was intentionally brief and very general. The reader is referred to Prigatano[11] and Sohlberg and Mateer[12] for comprehensive discussions of cognitive rehabilitation. In the clinical practice setting, consulting with a clinical neuropsychologist familiar with rehabilitation strategies can be extremely beneficial to the patient, in terms of enhancing their quality of life and in alleviating the fears/concerns of their caregivers. However, cognitive therapy must have a theoretical basis, and the provider should have a clear understanding of normal and impaired brain functions. In order to be most effective and efficient, treatment plans should be individualized for the patient, with realistic and attainable goals agreed upon by the patient, their caregivers, and the therapist.

Conclusions

The cognitive and behavioural changes that frequently accompany the diagnosis and treatment of a brain tumour are secondary to a complicated interaction of disease-, treatment-, and patient-related influences. In some case, these changes can be managed with relatively simple techniques. In other cases, it may be necessary to help patients come to terms with the permanent changes (cognitive and social) associated with brain cancer.

References

1 Hom, J. and Reitan, R. M. (1984). Neuropsychological correlates of rapidly vs. slowly growing intrinsic cerebral neoplasms. *J Clin Neuropsychol* **6**, 309.

2 DeWinter, A. E., Meyers, C. A., Hannay, H. J. *et al.* (1996). The effect of brain tumour growth rate on neuropsychological test performance. *J Int Neuropsychol Soc* **2**, 65.

3 Pavol, M. A., Meyers, C. A., Rexer, J. L. *et al.* (1995). Pattern of neurobehavioural deficits associated with interferon-alfa therapy for leukemia. *Neurology* **45**, 947–50.

4 Meyers, C. A., Schiebel, R. S., and Forman, A. D. (1991). Persistent neurotoxicity of systemically administered interferon-alpha. *Neurology* **41**, 672.

5 Meyers, C. A., Obbens, E. A. M. T., Scheibel, R. S. *et al.* (1991). Neurotoxicity of intra-ventricularly administered alpha-interferon for leptomeningeal disease. *Cancer* **68**, 88.

6 Meyers, C. A. and Yung, W. K. A. (1993). Delayed neurotoxicity of intra-ventricular interleukin-2, A case report. *J Neurooncology* **15** (3), 265–7.

7 Lewis, D. A. and Smith, R. E. (1983). Steroid induced psychiatric syndromes. *J Affect Disord* **5**, 319.

8 Kaufman, D. M. (1995). *Clinical neurology for psychiatrists* (4th edn), pp.239–41. W. B. Saunders Company, Philadelphia.

9 Meador, K. J. and Baker, G. A. (1997). Behavioural and cognitive effects of lamotrigine. *J Child Neurol* **12** (Suppl 1), S44–7.

10 Meyers, C. A., Weitzner, M. A., Valentine, A. D. *et al.* (1998). Methylphenidate therapy improves cognition, mood, and function of brain tumour patients. *J Clin Oncol* **16** (7), 2522–7.

11 Prigatano, G. P. (1999). *Principles of neuropsychological rehabilitation.* Oxford Univeristy Press, New York.

12 Sohlberg, M. M. and Mateer, C. A. (2001). *Cognitive rehabilitation, an integrative neuropsychological approach.* The Guilford Press, New York.

Chapter 6

Family care whilst the patient is attending the oncology centre

Linda Launchbury and Annette Landy

Introduction

Primary and secondary brain tumours can affect patients' physical, emotional, social, and cognitive abilities, and lead to personality and mood changes. Family care for people with tumours of the CNS is particularly important because the patient will frequently develop profound physical disabilities in combination with a marked deterioration of psychological, social, and cognitive functioning. The possibility of deterioration in intellect and personality is often the reason why intra-cranial malignancy is a particularly feared disease.

People with intra-cranial tumours often become frustrated by their dependence on others, and carers may become physically and emotionally exhausted and socially isolated whilst looking after a family member with this disease. Both carers and patients may sometimes discourage visitors, as they may be embarrassed, even ashamed, about the changes in their own (or their relative's) behaviour and want friends to remember them as they were. The change in the patient's personality may stop them being the loving and supportive partner they once were, or exaggerate their worst characteristics leading to increasing loneliness for all parties. Both the patient and their family have to adapt to an uncertain future and, in the case of high-grade astrocytomas, a short life-expectancy for the patient. Other people, with less aggressive tumours, may survive for many months, even years, becoming more and more disabled: this often has profound effects on family life. For these people the disease has many of the same effects as any chronic neurological condition.

Knowledge of the clinical effects of the intra-cranial malignancy and understanding the distress caused by the social and emotional changes this disease may cause, enables the specialist team to prepare the family and other carers for what may come, and to provide timely care and support, thus enabling the patient and family to have the best possible quality of life.

This chapter is concerned with the patient and family whilst the patient is being treated at an oncology centre, and does not consider the problems of chronicity. The authors aim to identify common causes of patient and family distress, and offer practical advice on how the effects of these can be minimized.

For the sake of brevity, the term 'family' also refers to friends and significant others.

Sources of evidence

A literature search using CINAHL and OVID databases showed over 10 000 articles concerned with family support—less than 10 of these dealt specifically with patients who had a primary or secondary brain tumour.

The evidence for this chapter is based on a review of the available literature, the authors' experience: LL as a clinical nurse specialist in a hospital-based palliative care service in a cancer centre, and AL as psychological therapist within a palliative care psychological and family support service. In addition the authors have drawn on the experience of colleagues working in neuro-oncology.

Causes of patient/family distress

Cancer not only has an impact on the patient, but also on the lives of friends and family.[1] Anxiety, distress, and depression in the patient may all be caused by the physical or psychosocial effects of brain tumours, including:

- the shock of the diagnosis, particularly when the patient has presented with only vague symptoms or with a very short history of any problems;
- a progressive loss of mobility;
- an awareness of a deterioration in their personal and social skills;
- an awareness of a deterioration in their thinking and reasoning skills— with a fear of 'going mad' or 'becoming demented';
- difficulty with communication from receptive or expressive dysphasia, for example, which is often intensely frustrating;
- fear, of having seizures, or shame if they do become a problem;
- bladder or bowel dysfunction;
- altered body image (e.g. facial swelling and weight gain from steroids, hair loss following radiotherapy, use of walking aids);
- the loss of independence;
- the loss of a future to look forward to;

- loss of role(s) and status, including the inability to work and earn money, the loss of roles as wife, mother, husband, father grandparent, and so on;
- the inability to drive;
- other complications associated with metastatic disease in people with secondary brain tumours, e.g. spinal cord compression.

The family often suffer extreme anxiety for all the reasons outlined above. In addition they have to witness the patient's deterioration and often feel powerless to help their distress, with which they have to live day and night. If the patient has deteriorated suddenly and rapidly, the family may be continually uneasy about what will happen next, and what they will have to cope with alone at home. They want to know what to do for the best. The family may be unable to relate to the patient who has undergone significant change in mood or personality and who may be, for example, venting anger and frustration aggressively or becoming disinhibited. The patient's dependence on the family can lead to the family members feeling isolated and unable to cope. If the patient was previously at work, there may also be financial difficulties, particularly if the patient was the main wage-earner.

All of these problems are common for patients with a primary or secondary brain tumour and they can be devastating.

Management

Such complex problems require a holistic approach, encompassing the psychological, social, spiritual, and physical aspects of care. Multidisciplinary teamwork is essential[1] but there should be a clear clinical leader. The person taking the leading role may change over the course of the disease; for example; from neuro-surgeon to neuro-oncologist to GP/family physician to palliative care specialist.

Whilst the patient and family are attending the oncology centre, distress can often be significantly reduced by promoting:

- open communication between patient, family, and health professionals;
- easy access to information about the disease and help that is available;
- psychological support for patient/family;
- effective discharge planning;
- rapid access to help at times of crises, through one agency—this may change over time from neuro-oncologist to GP/family physician to palliative care service;
- the provision of practical help;

- ensuring that the family physician/GP and nurses in the community know what is happening—they may have a long-standing relationship with the family and may be able to support the family even when the patient is in hospital and to care for the bereaved family in the longer term.

Open communication

Open communication between all parties enables individuals to discuss concerns freely and is encouraged by:

- Asking patients/family to outline their main concerns—particularly when a patient has an incurable high-grade glioma and where time may be very short.
- Involving both patient and family in decision-making at every stage.
- Good non-verbal communication, which should mirror what is being said verbally.[2] This avoids the possibility of giving 'mixed messages'. Communication is helped by, for example, attentive listening, good eye contact, and use of 'open questions'.
- Being approachable.
- Honesty without brutality.

The patient and family need to feel comfortable enough to ask any question. More importantly, clinicians need to take responsibility for giving patients and families opportunities to talk about sensitive areas that, although not mentioned by them, may be causing extreme anxiety. Examples include finding out if there have been changes in the patient's personality, if there are financial worries, or if the patient and family have concerns about current or feared intellectual deterioration.

Providing significant information

Patients and their families need easy and continuous access to information and health professionals should be prepared for this. In particular, information should automatically be given regarding:

- diagnosis: what it is, what it means and the implications;
- prognosis: explaining that there is always uncertainty around this issue;
- signs/symptoms: what they mean and the action that needs to be taken;
- planned investigations;
- treatment options (e.g. radiotherapy, surgery);
- steroid therapy: dose titration/adverse effects;
- disease progression: what is likely to happen/who will be leading treatment;

- follow-up appointments: with whom, where they will be, their purpose and when they will be needed;
- how to get help between appointments for medical and psychosocial problems;
- what support is available for them in the community.

The patient may want their partner or carer present when important news or information is given: the clinical team need to plan ahead in order to achieve this. Not only is this comforting to most patients but, in addition, if patients are unable to recall or comprehend information because of cognitive impairment, the family can reinforce it. Written information should be provided for the patient and family to refer to as they wish. The amount and depth of information given will depend upon the individuals concerned. If you are uncertain how much an individual or family want to know, use questions such as 'Are you the type of person that prefers to know all the facts?', 'Is there anything else you want to know?', 'Do you have all the information you need?'.

Repetition of information by different members of the team may be necessary, as many patients have memory loss or anxiety that prevents them from retaining information. Many people have difficulty hearing frightening news.

Many professionals find 'breaking bad news' difficult and distressing. This topic is not discussed in depth in this book, but many good texts are available. *Breaking bad news. A ten step approach* by Peter Kaye[3] is a practical, concise guide for professionals wishing to enhance their skills in this area. There are many good training courses available.

The ability to communicate effectively and humanely is increasingly recognized as one of the most important clinical skills that all clinicians need in order to give the best care to their patients and families—this skill needs to be reviewed and renewed throughout a clinician's career.

Communication with children

It is essential to keep children informed about what is happening to their parent, grandparent, or other who is dear to them, and to answer their questions honestly as they arise. It is essential to find out their fears. It is not uncommon for parents (and other adults) to feel that by keeping unpleasant facts from their children, they are protecting them. Children, even the very young, can perceive that something very wrong is happening. If nothing is explained to them, they will have their own fantasies about what it is and these may be horrifying; they may even feel that they are the cause of the problem. For the same reason, children should not be prevented from visiting their relatives whilst they are in hospital. (They should not, of course, be coerced.) Children (and the relatives bringing them into hospital) may need preparation before, and accompanying during, a visit to a place like the intensive care unit, or if there has been a catastrophic change in their parents' condition, but it is important that they are not kept away.

Helping parents to talk to their own children about an illness that is terrifying for them as adults is also an important skill. There is not one way of telling 'bad news' and the information does not all have to be given on one occasion. In general, formal 'set pieces' are best avoided. Parents may want a clinician present sometimes when talking to their children to help answer the medical questions, or they may chose to answer questions as they arise at home. Both parents and clinicians are often surprised by what children do already know, or have perceived for themselves, and may feel intimidated by the directness of children's questions.

All parents suffer unbearable pain at the prospect of separating from their children and anxiety about what will happen to the family when they have died. Helping them to prepare for this by the use of memory boxes, for example, and making practical arrangements for the children, as well as talking to them about what is going to happen, can go some way to alleviating this and to giving the children important helpful memories of this time. Any parent affected by personality change or cognitive deterioration in a partner can find it a relief to explain to children that this is a result of the illness and that mummy or daddy is still the same person underneath.

By involving the children in what is happening at every stage of their parent's illness and helping them with their grief, long-term psychological problems can be reduced. By supporting parents in talking to their children about what is happening in a way that is appropriate for their age, family unity can be enhanced and family stress reduced. Although this cannot be discussed in depth in this chapter, the care of children is central to palliative care. In many cases this work does not require specialist psychological intervention but is part of the normal care of families carried out by the multidisciplinary team, often by clinical nurse specialists, or palliative care social workers. Sometimes, particularly if there were difficulties before the illness, specialist family work will be required.

Legal problems

There may be medico-legal problems thrown up by illness, particularly intra-cranial malignancy that may cause cognitive deterioration. The advice of a solicitor and/or specialist social worker may be needed to help with:

- Arranging an appropriate form of power of attorney when a patient is no longer able to manage their own financial affairs—it may simply allow the family to use assets that are necessary for everyday expenses or may be necessary to prevent financial abuse of a vulnerable person.

- To ensure that a will is made correctly—patients should be encouraged to think about this early in their illness ('hope for the best and prepare for the worst'), whilst they have full mental faculties. Not everyone will become cognitively impaired but it is not always possible to predict who is going to be affected by this and unexpected physical deterioration is always possible.

- To help sort out the care of dependents—some elderly patients may be the sole carer of, for example, a middle-aged child with learning disability. Such parents suffer enormous anxiety about their child's existence after their death. Making provision can go some way to alleviating this. The children of divorced parents (where there is no continuing contact) will also need to be provided for.

Anticipating and offering skilled, qualified help to manage these issues is part of good family and palliative care.

Emotional and psychological support in family care

Holistic care has already been defined, as the integration of psychological, social, physical, and practical support. It can be seen from Fig. 6.1 that there is an enormous range of psychological and practical issues for anyone facing a life-threatening illness. In addition, the patient and family may have to deal with a bewildering number of healthcare professionals, machines, and treatments.

For a person with cognitive impairment and fear of future deterioration, this may result in much confusion and anxiety.

Why is there a need for emotional and psychological support?

A number of different studies over many years have shown that between 15% and 30% of people with life-threatening illness exhibit emotional and psychological distress serious enough to warrant professional intervention at some stage of their illness. Figures for family members are comparable. In addition, other studies have documented high levels of marital, sexual, and family problems associated with diagnosis of life-threatening illness and its treatment.

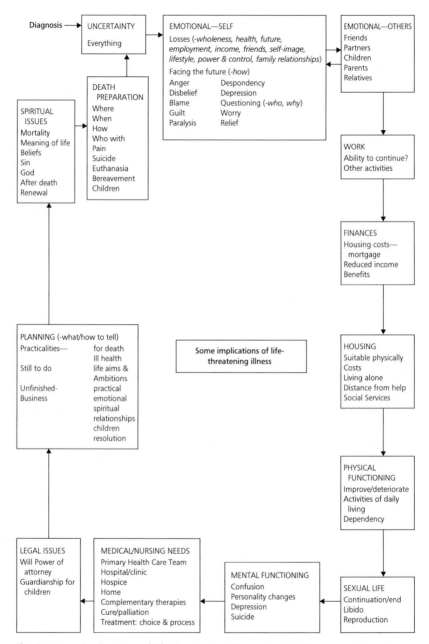

Fig. 6.1 Some implications of life-threatening illness. Carol Holloway and Annette Landy, 1991.

There are a number of simple psychological interventions that have been shown to be effective in reducing psychological distress for the majority of people with life-threatening illness. Clinicians working in oncology departments need to have these basic psychological skills in order to integrate emotional and psychological care for patients and families with excellent medical care.

Physical treatments are often extremely unpleasant. Some people refuse recommended physical therapies because of debilitating side-effects and fear of pain. Excellent symptom control can lead to better compliance with treatment, and reduced psychological and physical morbidity in both patient and family.

Pain management is a good example of where the physical and emotional aspects of the symptom are very strongly entwined. Managing all the facets of an individual's pain is likely to give a far better outcome than concentrating on physical symptoms alone.

The diagnosis of a brain tumour is often devastating emotionally for the patient and the family. The term 'death from diagnosis' has been used to describe the phenomenon that some relatives describe: they feel they lose their partner (or other relative) when personality change or cognitive deterioration takes place. If a high level of psychological awareness is present in all members of the team, these difficult issues can be managed sensitively throughout the time that a patient is being investigated and treated.

The effects of inevitable distress can be reduced rather than exacerbated if a thread of psychological care runs through the patient's management—which also embraces the family.

What is psychological support?

It cannot be overemphasized that excellent holistic care must encompass good emotional and psychological support. This is the remit for all members of the multidisciplinary team but wherever possible, specialized psychological assessments and interventions are best made by a 'customized' psychological or psycho-oncology service. Their expertise can attend to the most complex emotional and psychological needs of the patient, family and health care professional alike.

In accordance with recommendations from NHS Cancer Plans and the *Improving supportive and palliative care for adults with cancer* draft document (2002), a five-level model of psychological support has been developed as a basis for working with patients and their families (Table 6.1).

Table 6.1 A five-stage model of psychological support for working with patients and families

Level 0	Self-help and user groups
Level 1	Effective information-giving, communication, and general psychological care (given by all of the multidisciplinary team).
Level 2	Crisis management and simple psychological interventions (given by all of the multidisciplinary team).
Level 3	Counselling and psychotherapy, formal and specialist psychological support (given by counsellors and psychological therapists).
Level 4	Psychiatric and specialized medical psychotherapeutic interventions given by a range of psychological therapists e.g. clinical psychologists, psychiatrists, medical psychotherapists, counsellor, and others.

Continual psychological awareness in the multidisciplinary team may well prevent a whole range of problems, or lead to the early detection and better management of them. This awareness in the team and access to specialised psychological skills will help to:

- encourage patients to express any concerns, thus enabling and supporting their own problem-solving skills—many people have successfully coped with crises in their lives before and need help only in rediscovering confidence in their own ways of dealing with difficulties;

- enable patient and family to make adjustments to the diagnosis and to changing symptoms in the course of the illness;

- address the distress that may be associated with medical procedures, e.g. fear of needles, nausea and vomiting at the thought of chemotherapy, fear of radiotherapy, etc.;

- detect and manage anxiety and depression;

- manage disinhibited behaviour;

- manage aggressive behaviour in patients and members of the family;

- detect and relieve stressful obsessive and/or compulsive thoughts and/or actions;

- address fears about the future;

- elicit suicidal feelings and give any necessary help;

- enable patients to make necessary choices about treatments and changes in their way of life;

- address family problems and unhelpful dynamics, as well as supporting children in the family;

- address marital, sexual, and relationship problems;
- promote discussion of the ethical and moral dilemmas that arise when managing life-threatening incurable illness, e.g. when to stop disease-focused treatment;
- promote rehabilitation, both physical and psychological, so that patients can make the best use of any response to treatment;
- help patients and families acquire new skills and strategies for dealing with stress and worry, e.g. relaxation techniques;
- address quality of life issues, i.e. what is important to patients and families, what do they want treatment to achieve;
- manage grief reactions in illness and death;
- enable patients to explore the spiritual/religious meaning of what is happening.

When is psychological support needed?

A psychological thread of care needs to run though the management of all patients and families. Members of the specialist team need to be able to detect signs of psychological distress and have the ability to intervene appropriately—referring onto specialist services where this is needed.

Who can give psychological support?

All members of the multidisciplinary team will be able to offer support up to and including level 2 (see Table 6.1) and some will be able to work at level 3. Personnel suitable for delivering specialist psychological assessments and interventions include psychiatrists, medical psychotherapists, clinical psychologists, health psychologists, and recognized counsellors (Fig. 6.2).

Where there is no specialist service available, then consultancy or liaison with mental health teams may be able to provide some support, supervision and further training of the multidisciplinary team in psychological thinking.

How is psychological support given?

Definitions of psychological interventions:

Informal. Any psychological intervention offered as the need arises as part of a routine interaction. The practitioner may not have extended training in psychological interventions, but would normally have some clinical experience of dealing with psychological problems. It is part of the overall service offered by any member of the multidisciplinary team and is not offered separately.

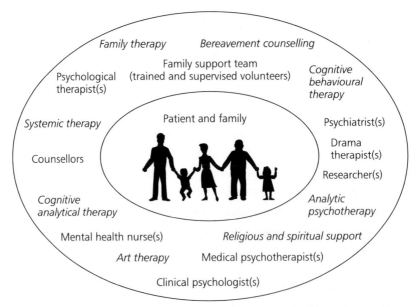

Fig. 6.2 Possible components of a psychological support service in oncology and palliative care.

Formal. A complete psychological treatment intervention offered as a series of set sessions, following a psychological assessment that generates a therapeutic plan. The practitioner will be sufficiently skilled to carry through a therapeutic intervention based on known theoretical frameworks.

Patients and families may sometimes decline referral to a psychological specialist outside the team they know—they may feel judged as being inadequate psychologically ('not a coper') or 'mentally ill'. People with intra-cranial malignancy may feel particularly vulnerable to these feelings because the disease affects the brain. These problems can often be avoided if the psychological therapist is a full member of the oncology or palliative care team, so that joint consultations are possible. Psychological therapists can also then offer indirect care to patients and families by supervising the psychological care given by another member of the team when direct consultations are not possible.

Summary of psychological care

There are many ways in which psychological care can help patients and families, and the neuropsychological complications that patients may develop are discussed in detail in Chapter 5. A psychologically informed approach to family care with specialist interventions, where needed, can help throughout the cancer journey.

By contributing to the psychological understanding of the issues raised by the diagnosis and treatment of brain tumours, assessments and interventions can be carried out to relieve psychological symptoms at any stage of the illness and in bereavement.

Specific problems are often associated with particular types of brain tumours—cognitive impairment, aggression, and disinhibition are often very difficult to manage. They also impose burdens for carers both family and professional. Adequate support is vital if these problems are to be contained for the well-being of all concerned.

The psychological service can have other roles:

supporting members of the multidisciplinary team in supervision and the provision of good psychological care of themselves;

taking part in case discussions about patients and families with particularly difficult problems;

offering consultation to healthcare staff encompassing the cognitive, emotional, behavioural, and social aspects of disease related issues.

Many patients will be receiving both disease-focused treatment and palliative care simultaneously. In order to maximize support, liaison and integrated working between the acute, palliative, and community sectors is essential. The patient and family will receive what they need from each service wherever they are; for example, patients may benefit from the rehabilitation that hospice out-patient and day therapy can offer or radiotherapy in the oncology centre.

Whilst it may not be possible to provide the kind of service outlined in, for example, the UK NHS Cancer and Supportive Care Plans, multidisciplinary teams will have access to training in communication skills, basic psychological assessments, and simple management techniques for relaxation and anxiety reduction.

Case studies

The following two case studies offer some insight into the benefits of combining physical care and psychological intervention. By addressing fully the psychological complexities and sometimes 'bizarre' behaviour of patients with brain tumours, the rest of the multidisciplinary team may use their time effectively to manage physical symptoms without the stress of also having to manage issues stemming from continuing challenging behaviour.

Case study 1: Janet

History

At the time of referral, Janet (aged 38) had been ill for 3 years with a brain tumour. She was married to Bill (aged 50) and they had two children—Darren 14 years old and Kylie, 8 years old. They lived on a low income, but by constant struggling, they continued to manage. Janet's physical condition was deteriorating. Having been a pretty and vivacious woman, she had become very overweight, bald, disinhibited, often confused, and very unsteady on her feet, and prone to falling over and 'fitting'. She attended the oncology department regularly and continued to have a variety of treatments. Despite being told that these treatments were palliative, both she and Bill were still hopeful that there would be a miracle cure. As her condition deteriorated, Bill found it harder to cope and he was sometimes tearful when speaking with oncology staff. As a result, Bill was offered some psychological support to 'help him cope and feel less depressed'. He presented as an exhausted, sad man. Both children were 'acting out' in school and Darren had started to play truant.

Interventions

After assessment, Bill was offered family support, a therapist for himself and Janet, and another therapist for the children. Some sessions were conducted together and some separately.

Janet had become 'paranoid' about people talking behind her back and did not allow Bill to do anything without her. As she gradually came to trust the team, she agreed to attend the Palliative Care Day Therapy Centre, in order to develop a social life with others in a similar predicament, and to be the recipient of various complementary therapies, mental stimulation, and good company. This left her husband free to have time out for him and his own psychotherapy sessions.

Issues that emerged from his sessions allowed Bill to look at:

- the emotional and practical losses he had suffered since Janet's illness;
- feelings of frustrated manhood;
- how to speak with the children;
- space to think and to plan for the future deterioration of Janet and her death;
- bereavement care for himself and his children.

One of the most important themes that emerged, was Bill's feeling of inadequacy and shame, as he was illiterate and of low intelligence. He had worked very hard and diligently all his life to achieve a reasonable standard of living, and

Janet had aided him in this by looking after all paperwork and bills, and helping the children with their homework. He willingly accepted a family support team volunteer to help him with these areas.

Issues that emerged with the children mostly centred on mixed feelings about their home situation.

Fear. Both children were scared of finding Janet dead or in some 'nasty' situation. Indeed, Darren had once found her unconscious, doubly incontinent, and 'sitting' on the kitchen floor whilst his father was shopping at the local supermarket.

Shame. He had also been embarrassed and consequently bullied at school, 3 years previously, after his mother came to collect him. On a number of occasions she had 'made an exhibition of herself' by speaking inappropriately or falling over. The worst occasion was when she walked across the playground laughing maniacally with a very unsteady gait—fell over and her wig rolled off in front of his best friend's mother.

Precocious behaviour. Kylie was not bothered by her mother's behaviour, but encouraged by Janet, she wore makeup and very unsuitable clothing for her age. Her command of swear words and rude comments was extensive.

Results

The provision of intensive therapeutic sessions provided time, space, and regularity for exploration and resolution of the issues presented above. It also allowed 'follow through' during the rest of Janet's illness, and this was integrated with the physical care being provided by the rest of the healthcare professional team. It allowed a shift in thinking and planning for Bill; a time for processing and moving on for the children; and was an opportunity for anticipatory grief before Janet's death.

Conclusion

Pre-death issues were either resolved or considerably lessened. After Janet had died, there was a much less complex bereavement reaction from both husband and children than might have been originally expected. This was due, at least in part, to the psychological interventions that were carried out using psychodynamic techniques together with practical problem-solving.

Case study 2: Robert

History

Robert (aged 35) was married to Beth (aged 33), and they have one child, John, aged six months.

Bob, a successful civil servant, had been ill for one year and was deteriorating rapidly. Over the last few months he had become confused, cognitively impaired, disinhibited, and rowdy. He had been verbally abusive to, and sexually disinhibited with, any passing woman. He masturbated publicly and often. On admission to hospital for symptom control, staff felt unable to manage him, and there was much embarrassment and anxiety about addressing the problems.

Supervision issues

The nursing team brought the issue to their session with the supervising psychological therapist, who enabled them to explore ways of understanding and solving these sensitive problems.

Interventions

Nurses 'role played' different ways of approaching the subject with Beth. In reality they found Beth was similarly embarrassed and relieved to share her concerns. Once the problem was openly talked about, the difficulties lessened. There were direct conversations with Bob and, although he did not seem to understand them fully, the suggestions made to him led to a significant change in his behaviour. He became quieter and did not masturbate publicly. Speaking simply, kindly, and yet authoritatively, he 'relearned' appropriate social skills.

Results

Beth is now able to enjoy a family social life, often going on excursions with him and the baby without mishap. The anxiety that surrounded the situation has continued to be much reduced. With occasional reinforcement, and gentle encouragement, Bob has continued to behave in a much more acceptable way.

Beth has adapted to the situation by accepting that she has 'lost' her husband as an equal partner and has learned to relate to him in an almost maternal way. She says, 'I have two children to look after now . . .'

Conclusions

This case shows the benefit of a short but defined psychological intervention based on cognitive-behavioural lines for Robert, together with brief focal psychotherapy for Beth to enable her grief to be shown for the loss of a 'normal' marriage and family future, and adaptation to recognizing and resolving issues arising from inappropriate behaviour.

The final benefit was that this episode boosted the confidence of the nursing team in 'communication and problem-solving'. Rather than avoiding an embarrassing and worsening situation, the team sensitively worked together in a group-supervision session, to produce a successful strategy that improved the outcome for the patient and family and reduced everybody's levels of stress and anxiety.

Discharge-planning

Many neuro-oncology patients and their families express concern about how they will cope at home. Common fears include managing the physical care of the patient, and adapting to inevitable deterioration and short life-expectancy. For in-patients, early discharge planning is essential to allay such fears and prevent unnecessary delays, and to facilitate a smooth transition from hospital. Although the majority of patients want to go home and to die at home,[1] it cannot be assumed that this is the aim of every individual or their family. Adequate support may not be available.

Care options must be discussed openly with patient and family in order for an informed choice of placement to be made. Placement for this group of patients is often difficult. In most areas the care options are:

- home with all support and care that is available—often this is less than is needed;
- residential/nursing home;
- continuing care/palliative care bed e.g. in community hospital.

Dunlop[1] maintains that patients and families can overcome uncertainty and fear in order to remain at home during a terminal illness.

Practical positive help offered by physiotherapists and occupational therapists is essential. They will assess what the patients can do, what will help them to do more, and what the family need at home in order to give the best chance that a discharge will be successful.

As well as advising on changes to the environment, it can be a great boost to a patient's morale (and therefore the family's) if the patient can be helped to be as physically independent as possible.

End-of-life planning

Many patients have strong opinions about where they want to be cared for and the degree of medical intervention that they want when they deteriorate, and who they would wish to act as proxy if decisions have to be made when they are no longer able to speak for themselves. These are often difficult topics for patients, families, and clinicians to address directly but it is important that patients are given the opportunity to express their views on these and other related subjects. Very few people have advanced directives and even those that have may not reveal them when they become seriously ill. Studies have shown that patients expect clinicians to initiate discussion on these areas—the timing of these conversations is crucial: too early and they may upset the patients' need to engage with treatment in a hopeful way, even if the treatment is palliative in intent; too late and the patient may not be able to participate in the decisions and there may not be time to put in place any arrangements that are necessary to achieve the patient's goals. Any team member, in a competent supportive team, who has full information, can start these conversations or respond to the patients' questions honestly when the time is right.

End-of-life care

The physical and psychosocial changes that accompany intra-cranial malignancy often restrict the choice of place in which patients can be given adequate care. The following are common limitations:

- hospices will often admit patients for a relatively short time only and may not have suitably qualified staff or facilities adapted to give safe care to patients with cognitive impairment or difficult personality changes;
- nursing homes are often unsuitable for young patients and are often frequently unable to care for those with cognitive impairment;
- a young, strong, disabled person with cognitive impairment may be difficult to care for at home, particularly if they have personality changes or if the partner has young children to care for as well;
- outside specialized psychiatric units, clinical staff may not have been trained to deal with aggression: a significant proportion of patients may develop disinhibition or aggression as the tumour progresses;
- many private nursing homes are unsuitable for physically disabled patients who have progressive disease—potential problems include falls and seizures;
- the staff of psychiatric wards often feel unable to manage the medical problems that affect patients with brain tumours.

This issue is of increasing concern because the number of people with intra-cranial malignancy is increasing. Some sort of medium term 'continuing care' facility would be ideal but there are few suitable units at present, and often a mixture of provision has to be found to prevent unbearable strain on the family or long-term admission to a neurosurgical or oncology ward, which may be far from home.

It is often extremely helpful for the patient and family to make links with the local hospice and community palliative care team early in the course of treatment at the oncology centre. As well as admitting patients for the control of difficult symptoms (rather than re-admitting to the acute centre), some hospices are able to support the family by offering respite care and day-centre places for the patient. Both of these options will give the family planned relief, which will enable them to cope with a difficult situation for longer. In addition, hospices often have family support and bereavement services, and can give other help for carers, e.g. volunteer sitters. The family can use these services locally, even if the patient is receiving in-patient care at an acute hospital some distance from home.

Anecdotal evidence suggests that patients with intra-cranial malignancy are more commonly admitted to hospices for end-of-life care than patient with other cancers. Some, unfortunately, deteriorate and die after weeks or months in a tertiary referral centre without ever being discharged.

Discharge home—what needs to be done?

Do:

- confirm that the patient and family both want discharge home;
- ensure that the primary care/community care team is fully informed about what is going on and are involved in the discussion of plans for future care;
- identify a co-ordinator responsible for all the practical aspects of discharge—it prevents confusion and either everything being done twice or not being done at all;
- involve the patient and family: sometimes there will be differences of opinion between them about what is needed—separate sensitive discussions may be required;
- ensure that they have all the information they want (and again needs may be different) about diagnosis, prognosis, and likely disease progression;
- ensure that patient and family are aware of support they will have, any other services that may be useful, and how to contact these services;
- ensure that the family know whom to contact in an emergency;
- consider arranging regular planned, respite care.

Do not:

- assume all patients want to go home;
- make promises of care in the community without confirming its availability.

Who needs to be involved?

A smooth discharge home is dependant upon good communication between the patient, family, and all professionals involved, and especially hospital and community services. Table 6.2 gives suggestions of the professionals who may

Table 6.2 Professionals who may be involved in discharging a patient

Who needs to be involved?	Why?
G.P./Family Physician	Update re: diagnosis, prognosis, patient/family understanding, current health status, treatment plan, medications, etc. Medical care at home and after care of family.
District Nurse/Community Nurses	Update as above; assessment of nursing needs. e.g. dressings, syringe driver etc.; support of patient and family.
Occupational Therapist	Assessment of activities of daily living; provision of aids e.g. commode, handrails.
Physiotherapist	Assessment of mobility; aids e.g. frame.
Social Services	Assessment of care; meals on wheels; financial benefits.
Hospital Support Nurse (neuro-oncology/oncology)	Support/information; symptom control.
Palliative Care Team/Nurse	Support/information; symptom control; introduction to community palliative care services.
Psychologist/Counsellor	Psychological support patient/family.
Speech Therapist	Dysphasia—assess/advise.
Dietician	Nutrition—assess/advise.
Chaplain/Minister of Religion	Spiritual support.

Consider:
- hospital at home
- day centre
- respite care
- sitting service e.g. crossroads

Support Groups (see below)	To assist patient/family to cope at home.

When children involved, consider:

• Health Visitor	Additional support for children
• School Nurse/Counsellor	
• Teacher	

Complicated Discharges:
- Discharge liaison Team
- Family Meeting/Case Conference
- Consider phased discharge (home for a day, weekend, initially)

be involved. The list is not exhaustive and will vary depending upon the individual needs of the patient/family.

Case study

Mr A was 40 years old, married with an 18-month-old child. He was recently diagnosed with a primary brain tumour and had debulking surgery followed by radiotherapy. Discharge home had been planned and subsequently postponed at the request of the family several times. Mr A became anxious at the delay in discharge. Ward staff were unsure if the family actually wanted to take Mr A home.

A case conference was arranged and attended by the patient's wife and parents, occupational therapist, physiotherapist, ward nurse and discharge liaison nurse. It emerged that the family were extremely anxious about how they would cope at home. Mrs A suffered from M.E. and did not drive. She was unsure that she would be able to manage her husband and the young child.

A plan was agreed of the necessary care and support the family would need. This included:

- Mr A's parents offering to sit with Mr A on a regular basis and to take Mrs A shopping weekly;
- occupational therapy three times/week;
- day centre weekly;
- respite care booked for 6 weeks after discharge;
- community Macmillan (palliative care) Nurse visits to support Mr A/family;
- regular contact with GP/family physician and District Nurse.

Mr A was discharged several days later. Since discharge, the family have cancelled attendance at the day centre, as they were managing well and felt it was no longer necessary.

'Caring for the carers'

Supporting distressed patients and carers through the palliative phase of illness can be challenging and emotionally stressful for health professionals and can lead to 'burnout'. Support, education, and clinical supervision are recommended. A psychotherapist is an invaluable team member, though often not available in acute trusts. Many patients with primary or secondary brain tumours need palliative care from diagnosis. Cure may not be an option. Health professionals may feel helpless—that there is little that can be done to ease the patient/family's suffering. The emphasis here is on helping patients achieve the best possible quality of life through:

- good symptom control; rehabilitation where possible;
- addressing psychological, spiritual, and social concerns;
- helping both patient and family adapt to an uncertain future;
- supporting difficult choices, e.g. where to die.

Finally, health professionals can be a support to the patient and family by simply continuing to maintain contact throughout the terminal stage. This reassures patients and their families that they have not been abandoned. Attributed to Hippocrates:[4]

- To cure occasionally,
- to relieve often,
- to comfort always.

Support groups

BACUP
3 Bath Place, Rivington Street, London EC2A 3JR
tel: 020 7696 9003
www.cancerbacup.org.uk

Brain Tumour Foundation
PO Box 162, New Malden, Surrey KT3 4WH
tel: 0208336 2020
btf.uk@virgin.net

UK Brain Tumour Society
BAC House, Bonehurst Road, Horley, Surrey RH6 8QG
tel: 01293 781479
info@braintumour.org

References

1   **Dunlop, R.** (1998). *Cancer, palliative care.* Springer, London.
2   **Lugton, J.** (2002). *Communicating with dying people and their relatives.* Radcliffe Medical Press Ltd, Abingdon.
3   **Kaye, P.** (1996). *Breaking bad news. A ten-step approach.* EPL Publications, London.
4   **Barnes, P.** (1988). To comfort always. *BMJ* **297**, 631.

Further reading

British Psychological Society Division of Clinical Psychology (1997). *A guide for purchasers of clinical psychology services (oncology).* British Psychological Society.

DoH (2000). *NHS cancer plan.* DoH, London.

DoH (2000). *Treatment choice in psychological therapies and counselling. Evidence based guidelines.* DoH, London.

Harrison, J., Haddad, P., and Maguire, P. (1995). The impact of cancer on key relatives, a comparison of relative and patient concerns. *Eur J Cancer* **31A**, 1736–40.

Hoskin, P. and Makin, W. (1998). *Oncology for palliative medicine.* Oxford University Press, Oxford.

Meyer, T. J. and Mark, M. (1995). Effects of psychosocial interventions with cancer patients, a meta-analysis of randomised experiments. *Health Psychology* **14**, 101–8.

National Institute for Clinical Excellence (NICE). (2004). *Guidance on cancer services— improving supportive and palliative care for adults with cancer.* NICE Cancer Service Guidance. National Institute for Clinical Excellence, London. Available from www.nice.org.uk.

Chapter 7

Acquired communication and swallowing difficulties in patients with primary brain tumours

Helen White

This chapter discusses some of the issues and complexities involved for those people diagnosed with a primary brain tumour who have developed communication and/or swallowing difficulties.

The multi faceted nature of cancer and its treatment frequently requires a complex management process that involves many different professionals and different modalities of treatment. For the patient with acquired communication and/or swallowing disorders caused by a primary brain tumour, this process can be helped to run as smoothly as possibly by early recognition of such problems and referral to a specialist speech and language therapist.

In the United Kingdom, primary brain tumours occur in approximately six people per 100 000 per year.[1]

This chapter describes the role of the speech and language therapist working with the disorders of communication and swallowing as part of the multi professional neuro-oncology team. It does not cover the speech and language therapy management of paediatric tumours, nor does it provide detailed definitions and in-depth descriptions of speech, language, and swallowing disorders. There are many books dedicated to this purpose, e.g. Darley, Aronson, and Brown,[2] Duffy,[3] Logemann,[4] Murdoch,[5,6] Sullivan and Guilford.[7]

The specialist hospital environment

An inherent danger for a clinician who works solely within an oncology setting is to forget the fear that the word 'cancer' generates amongst most people. Perhaps especially 'brain tumours', which threatens the personality and intellect as well as the body. This fear seems to cross cultural and social boundaries with ease. So, it is an ongoing challenge for the professional to remain mindful of the powerful impact a diagnosis of cancer can have upon the patient, their family, and friends. Pound et al.[8] discuss models of disability and the media's representation of heroic battles fought against illness. They refer to studies in narrative medicine that highlight the fact that, while the disease or illness may follow standard physiological forms, personal experiences are not homogenous.[8] Apart from the diverse, idiosyncratic interpretations of illness, Frank[9] and Greenhalgh and Hurwitz[10] illustrate the important influences and expectations of institutional and practitioner cultures.

The medical environment of a hospital can be imbued with a sense of the power of science to offer a cure. Frank[9] describes the 'restitution' narrative, where the specialist professional can be perceived as the expert and the patient the tragic or long-suffering victim. Attached to the title of 'expert' are expectations. One expectation can be to have answers to all questions. It can feel very uncomfortable not to have the answer. When you do, it may contain information the patient, and/or their family, do not want to hear. As a specialist speech and language therapist working within a neuro-oncology team in a cancer hospital, I frequently bear witness to, discuss and feel challenged by experiencing, this discomfort.

The multi-professional team

Multidisciplinary teamwork is the cornerstone of rehabilitation therapy.[11] The many and varied problems experienced by patients with brain tumours and their caregivers, mean their needs are more likely to be met by the diverse skills from a variety of professions. There is a potential risk of fragmentation of patient services. The ethic of collaborative working is essential for effective team intervention. The full range of relevant disciplines needs to be involved for comprehensive and effective management.[12] However, the dynamics of teamwork can be complex and challenging. There may be differing professional ideologies and approaches; for example, the pathophysiological versus a holistic, problem-solving approach.[11]

A multi-professional team in which people are supportive and respectful of each other's professional roles, and where information is shared and management options discussed, directly improves the quality of care that is given to the patient. Teamwork implies co-operation and the characteristics of a team can be summarized by:[12,13]

- shared goals
- interdependence
- co-operation
- co-ordination of activities
- task specialization

- division of effort
- mutual respect.

Professional team members may be involved at different stages of the illness. They need to be aware of their clinical responsibility and accountability within the continuum of the patient's care.

The patient and their family hold a pivotal role within the team. The diagnosis of a malignant brain tumour is a potent agent for disrupting their pattern of life. Their lives are now defined by uncertainties and continual change. The patient and their family's perceptions, priorities, and preferred methods of dealing with their disease need to be heard and respected.[14,15]

Localization

Communication and swallowing are neurological functions. The speech and language therapist is concerned with specialist assessment and management of disorders of these vital functions. The complications of primary intra-cranial tumours of the dominant cerebral hemisphere and posterior fossa frequently initiate a referral to the speech and language therapist. These tumours may affect the functions of speech, language, and swallowing.

Language

The majority of right-handed people are left-hemisphere dominant for language. While it is recognized that many areas of the brain are involved with language processing, and that different tracts have different roles, the complex relationship between structure and function is not fully understood.[16] The best-understood structures involved are the frontal, temporal, and parietal lobes of the cerebral cortex. The importance of the subcortical structures (thalamus and basal ganglia) and their function in language processing is increasingly acknowledged but is still ill-defined, especially when caused by brain tumours.[17] To add to this complexity, distortion and/or compression of the tumour can occur at a distance from the tumour. The consequent impairment (aphasia) may have no direct relationship with the location of the tumour.[6,18] Scheibal et al.[19] describe research yielding mixed findings on the relationship between tumour location and cognitive dysfunction.

Speech and swallowing

Primary brain tumours involving the ventricular system, brainstem, cerebellum, and cranial nerves may cause impairment(s) of speech (dysarthria) and/or swallowing (dysphagia).

Complicating factors for communication and swallow functions

Important factors that can contribute to the variety, level, type, and combination of communication and/or swallowing problems include:

- grading of the tumour;
- tumour recurrence, transformation, or progression;
- existence of surrounding oedema;
- previous treatment, e.g. surgery, radiotherapy;
- medication;
- other sequelae, e.g. epilepsy.

Not all primary brain tumours cause communication and/or swallowing difficulties. However, the likelihood of these occurring does increase when there is a combination of two or more treatment methods.[7]

Role of speech and language therapy

Core roles for the speech and language therapist when patients are referred to them diagnosed with malignant primary brain tumour, include:

- assessment and differential diagnosis;
- therapy, advice, and information;
- monitoring;
- referring on to local hospital and community services, as appropriate;
- ongoing support and reassurance by:
  - being available/accessible to patient and/or carers throughout the course of the disease;
  - being an advocate for the patient within the hospital setting;
  - suggesting or adapting practical compensatory strategies to support their changing communication status.

Communication

Kibler[20] quotes Rene Descartes (1596–1650) 'I think, therefore I am' to illustrate the value and importance of the human brain. It is the organ of the body that is, above all others, linked with our sense of self. Our purpose and meaning in the world is based on who we are and what we can do.

Speech and language shape our thoughts and dreams, and permit interaction with those people around us. Language is the currency of relationships,[21] and is intrinsic and essential to our well-being. Its value and complexity may not become apparent until it is disrupted.

When the diagnosis of a malignant brain tumour is combined with an acquired communication problem, the effect is often described as devastating. Not just by the patients but also by key people in their lives. Brain tumours may disrupt communication at any level. The disruption can range from occasional hesitation with word finding, to a severe loss of language across the expressive modalities of speaking and writing, and the receptive modalities of understanding speech and reading. The person becomes aphasic. In the United Kingdom, the commonest cause of aphasia is cerebrovascular accidents and, every year, at least 20 000 people become aphasic.[21] The experience for cancer patients may be very different, as they can expect deterioration rather than stability and improvement.

Language

Aphasia is a complex disorder of language processing that takes many forms. It may affect:[21]

- the ability to put ideas and intentions into spoken and written language;
- speaking in grammatical sentences;
- spelling and writing—dysgraphia;
- understanding what is written—dyslexia;
- understanding and using other forms of communication.

Other disorders, such as oral and verbal dyspraxia (disorder of motor speech programming where muscle strength is undiminished), and dyscalculia, may also be present.

Aphasia and primary brain tumours

There are important factors that differentiate management of the aphasia within this patient group from the management of the aphasia caused by a cerebrovascular accident or head injury. The speech and language therapist has to consider these factors when trying to support the patient's communication needs.

Prognosis When diagnosed with a high-grade aggressive primary brain tumour and a prognosis that may be measured in months, not years, the aphasic patient's focus is unlikely to be attending intensive language impairment-based therapy.

Fluctuations Aphasia caused by a malignant brain tumour will generally have a fluctuating but ultimately progressive pattern, which can be further complicated and compromised by many issues: the disease, its treatment, and the related side-effects. An example of a transient treatment side-effect of radio-therapy is somnolence.[22]

Barriers Further barriers impacting on cognition and language function may include:

- poor memory—delayed language processing can further compromise short term memory function;
- reduced concentration and short attention span—especially immediately post-surgery and during and after radiotherapy treatment, this can also impact on memory function;
- distractibility—increased sensitivity to background noise and visual distractions;
- generalized fatigue—the aphasic patient already needs extra energy to process language; it becomes too effortful to 'chat'; they need extra time to process and to respond.

Supporting communication

Referral to the speech and language therapist may be at any stage of the overall patient management. Key concepts of their intervention and management are governed by the disease and treatment factors, such as recurrence, surgery, radio-therapy treatment. It is essential we recognize that we are asking the aphasic patient to make sense of their disease and treatment options using the very medium that is damaged—language. As previously mentioned, language is necessary to make sense of or give meaning to our world.

The Patient A key intervention for the speech and language therapist is enabling and supporting the patient to understand their disease, and treatment and management options. To support the aphasic patient's communication needs there are individual issues to consider:

- the patient's reaction to the diagnosis and prognosis;
- the changing needs of patients' and carers' during the disease process;
- no offer of a 'cure';
- periods of no treatment, of being asked to 'watch and wait';
- possibility of tumour transformation, recurrence or progression;
- decisions about future treatment options;
- individual psychosocial needs;
- coping styles;
- previous life experiences;
- communication style and communication needs.

These individual differences are highly relevant and the therapist needs to be aware of their potential influence when meeting and assessing the patient's communication impairment. The timing of the intervention is paramount and will dictate the type of language assessment. The overall prognosis may be poor, thus precluding a lengthy formal language assessment. The previously mentioned factors may be contributing to fluctuating levels of communicative abilities within and between days. It can be difficult to identify a precise level of breakdown and limits the usefulness of assessment results. This can not only be challenging, but can also be a source of frustration for everyone involved. For example, the patient may be able to understand and answer multiple choice or open questions one day but only cope with closed questions the next.

Family, friends, and colleagues Modelling good supportive communication to family, friends, and work colleagues is another key role for the speech and language therapist.[23,24]

It is helpful if a speech and language therapist can attend the medical consultation. The focus will usually be on the disease and its complications, and yet by supporting communication with subtle changes we can enable the patient to participate more and reveal their competencies. To observe a patient's communication skills within a conversation, but without them being 'tested', can provide invaluable information for future intervention.

Initially the speech and language therapist can offer practical suggestions by identifying the barriers to effective communication and, with ongoing review, offer practical supportive strategies:

- be aware of where the aphasic patient is within their disease trajectory;
- minimize distractions;
- allow time, with a calm, friendly, encouraging approach;
- make sure the aphasic patient understands the purpose of the conversation;
- talk directly to the aphasic patient and ask them what is/is not helpful;
- have pen and paper for both people to use—writing or drawing can support what is being said;
- speech should be clear, slightly slower, and of normal volume;
- use straightforward language, avoiding jargon—the names of brain tumours or medication are inevitably long and complex but can be clearly written for future reference;
- say one thing at a time, and pause between these 'chunks' of information;
- structure questions carefully;

- regularly check that the patient understands;
- make it clear when there is a change of topic;
- support the spoken language with appropriate non-verbal communication;
- a written summary containing salient/key information is useful, especially when the information is new and complex, the patient and carers are anxious, or the memory function is known to be impaired.

If there is concern about sounding or appearing to be patronizing, it can help if you explicitly state your concern and ask the aphasic patient or their carers to let you know what is or is not helpful. This may (in some cases) improve their, and your, awareness and build upon their confidence to participate within consultations. Aphasic patients often describe other people's reactions to aphasia as being a potential barrier. The onus, or balance, of the conversation may have to change for it to be successful. The conversation partner may need to learn to develop skills to elicit and interpret the aphasic patient's communicative intent. These strategies can help to reduce any feelings of inadequacy or embarrassment for all concerned.[11]

Recommended practical resources for supported conversation and aphasia information are referenced.[21,25]

Communication aids

If there is a severe level of either expressive and/or receptive asphasia, or a severe level of dysarthria, augmentative or alternative communication (AAC) may be considered. This may range from basic picture charts or books, to electronic aids and computer programs. No matter how simple or sophisticated the aid, communication changes from a two-way to a three-way process. Motivation to communicate is paramount. After the speech and language therapist has assessed and identified the most appropriate ACC, it requires planning, extra concentration and time, listening, watching, and interpretation by both the patient and the conversation partner. Awareness of these factors facilitates more realistic expectations of the AAC, thus reducing any potential disappointment. Pound *et al.*[8] advocate the use of an individually negotiated life-book. This contains key events and information (written and pictorial) relating to the patient's life and can be used to explore, affirm, and provide concrete representation of their past and present. This could be integrated within the communication books or files, and highlights the links between identity, communication, and self-expression.[8]

Quality of life

Quality of life means different things to different people. The psychosocial effects of aphasia are intrinsically linked with quality of life issues for the aphasic patient and their family. Central to a speech and language therapist's role is not only to reveal the patient's communicative competencies to support and maintain the optimum level of communication, but also to elicit, acknowledge, and respect their priorities and key issues. It is vital to acknowledge the different coping styles and attitudes of the patient and the key people in their lives.[20,21] There will continue to be adjustments to make as the disease changes or progresses. For example, role changes within the family,[26,27] or in the work environment, facing their mortality. The aphasia may exacerbate any pre-existing difficulties in the patient's social life, employment, personal relationships, or psychological state. These will inevitably have an impact on their emotional and psychological well-being and self-image.[28]

Speech

Dysarthria is a neuromuscular disorder of speech caused by weakness or paralysis of the relevant muscles, i.e. muscles of respiration, phonation and articulation. The type of dysarthria reflects the lesion site and may present as a flaccid, spastic, ataxic, or mixed dysarthria. For example, an upper motor neuron or spastic dysarthria is characterized by slurred, imprecise, and effortful speech with a slowed rate.[2]

Again, the complex pattern and course of the brain disease, and its management, will influence the intervention. The pivotal aim is still to support the patient's optimum level of communication. While the therapy is essentially the same as for cranial nerve deficits of any other aetiology, the fluctuating abilities and treatment side-effects may again challenge the therapist by dictating a more flexible approach to therapeutic intervention. For example, a patient's radiotherapy treatment regimen may indicate that it is more appropriate to use an AAC *before* facilitating intelligible speech by encouraging oro-facial and articulatory exercises.

Aphasia case history—Rachel

Medical history and treatment In 1995 Rachel, 49, presented with a 5-year history of intermittent complex seizures. An MRI scan revealed a left tempero-parietal lesion and she underwent debulking surgery. Histology confirmed a grade III anaplastic astrocytoma. Rachel completed a 6-week course of radiotherapy treatment in November 1995.

Current status Annual MRI scans indicate stable disease. Symptons include intermittent headaches, left-sided inco-ordination, short-term memory deficits, and expressive aphasia characterized by mild word retrieval and writing impairments. Her medication includes carbemazepine and lamotrigine, and she has been seizure-free for 5 years.

Social history Rachel has a close, supportive family. She lives with her husband, their three children live and work away from home. Prior to her diagnosis she had worked as a librarian and was actively involved with local community and church activities. Rachel had a ready sense of humour, loved reading, and writing poetry. She took great pride in her communication skills and felt she made the most of her life.

Speech and language therapy intervention In January 1996 Rachel's hospital doctor referred her to SLT (speech and language therapy) having witnessed Rachel's obvious frustration with word-finding difficulties. Rachel became very distressed when the language assessments revealed both the severity of her word-retrieval problems, and her inability to generate written letters and words. She admitted to being aware of these deficits but had found it too upsetting, and refused to contemplate, coming to the hospital or being referred to a community SLT. A month later Rachel asked for a contract of SLT. She preferred her oncology care to be 'all under one house'. A 6-week contract of weekly out-patient therapy was negotiated. The focus was on written output, including home exercise programmes.

Initial therapy sessions involved Rachel's husband, and discussions included the nature of Rachel's aphasia in the context of her diagnosis and medical treatment. For example, the impact of somnolence on word-finding and consequent need to adapt learned strategies. Rachel relied on a symbol/alphabet chart to help with letter- and single-word recognition, as the conversion rules for sound/letter and letter/sound were impaired. Written output expanded from single words (crosswords, anagrams, synonyms) to phrases—written picture descriptions, writing postcards. Improvement was noted in her word-retrieval, and she was more ready to use other strategies when struggling to find a word. For example, describing it, drawing it, or, eventually, writing it down.

Rachel was highly motivated and assertive. She was intolerant of tasks that she perceived to be irrelevant to her needs. Luckily, she had previously been an avid diary keeper, letter writer, scrabble player, and had loved doing crosswords. At the end of the contract, although still needing the alphabet chart, she was writing at sentence level and keeping a daily journal. It was agreed that therapy would be 'indirect' and Rachel would write a monthly letter to the therapist (this still continues). Rachel's communication is scattered with occasional hesitancies, confusion with spatial words such as 'push/pull', muddling the letters w/m or p/b/d. She needs extra time to process the written word but is now reading books.

Current intervention Direct SLT follow-up occurs when Rachel attends medical out-patient appointments. She now reports to be unembarrassed by her mild word-finding 'hiccups'. Recently she successfully wrote, and read aloud, her church's annual report about their many charity events. Over the last 7 years, with the support of family and friends, and her own personal faith, Rachel appears to have developed a sense of identity that incorporates her medical diagnosis and the consequent impairments. She does not appear to be handicapped by these, and reports to value and love her current life.

Swallowing

When a dysphagic patient is referred to a speech and language therapist, the main purpose of their intervention is, where possible, to prolong safe and pleasurable oral intake, while optimizing nutrition and hydration.

Swallowing refers to the entire act of glutition from the moment food and drink is placed in the mouth, through the oral, pharyngeal, and oesophageal stages until it enters the stomach.[4] The swallow process, although rapid, is an extremely complex action involving voluntary and involuntary components. It requires intact anatomy, mucosa, six cranial nerves, brainstem, 34 skeletal muscles, striated and smooth muscles.[29] Any disruption of this anatomy or physiology may result in disordered swallowing—dysphagia.

Localization

The swallowing centre (medullary reticular formation) is located in the brainstem and acts as a neuronal pool organizing the synergy necessary for normal swallowing. The roles of the cerebellum and cortical input for controlling swallowing are less clear.[4]

As with communication disorders, swallowing difficulties may present at any point of the continuum of care for people diagnosed with primary brain tumours. Tumours may infiltrate or compress the brainstem affecting the corticobulbar tracts or medullary centre. Patients with large unilateral supratentorial tumours may present with dysphagia when there is a decreased level of consciousness and contralateral weakness of the tongue and face. The dysphagia often fluctuates varying in severity, complexity and frequency.[18]

Psychological impact

The psychological impact of dysphagia must not be underestimated. In Western society, eating and drinking are generally thought of as pleasurable social activities. Contrast this thought with dreading meal times, being too embarrassed to eat with your family in your own home, let alone eating out in restaurants. The humiliation and adjustment in having to rely upon others to feed you—probably for the first time since you were an infant. Dysphagic patients frequently describe the feelings of inadequacy, lack of control, changing body image, reduced confidence, low self-esteem, loss of dignity, fear, anger, and guilt.

Management issues

The speech and language therapist may be involved with swallowing management at any stage of the disease process, but an early referral is preferable. As previously mentioned, treatment and management can be complex. The dysphagic symptons may be new, ongoing, recurring, or progressing. The patient's prognosis may be short. Treatment may affect the severity or have an impact on the dysphagia. For example, chemotherapy treatment may be suppressing the immune system, so the dysphagic patient is less able to tolerate chest infections; steroids may increase the patient's appetite, so they find it difficult to follow suggested compensatory strategies that included taking small amounts and eating slowly. These issues highlight the importance of collaborative working within and between the hospital and community teams.

Assessment and management

It is the oro-pharyngeal stages of the swallowing process that are the focus of the speech and language therapist's intervention. There are two aspects of the dysphagia assessment that commonly cause confusion—the presence/absence of a reflex cough, and the role of the gag reflex in the swallowing process.

Reflex cough If a patient is not coughing after swallowing food or drink it is often assumed that they are safe to swallow. In fact, an absent cough reflex can mean that aspiration may be occurring silently. There is a high incidence of silent aspiration with neurogenic dysphagia.[18] Reflexive coughing associated with oral intake does indicate that the material has penetrated the laryngeal vestibule, reached the vocal cords, and their brisk adduction attempts to eject the material into the pharynx. It is a protective mechanism and provides a useful sign that the food or drink has started to go the 'wrong way'. This contrasts with not coughing, which may have more serious consequences.

The role of the gag reflex The gag is triggered by noxious substances, such as vomit or reflux, and aims to squeeze the material up and out of the pharynx. This contrasts with the swallow's well-organized set of motor actions that aim to take the food/drink safely and efficiently from mouth to stomach.[4] Many individuals who have normal swallowing abilities demonstrate reduced or absent gag reflexes. There is little data to support that the presence or absence of a gag reflex in a neurologically dysphagic patient has any relationship with their ability to swallow.[30] The presence or absence of a patient's gag reflex does not predict their ability to swallow safely.

Assessment

Dysphagia assessment necessitates a careful bedside evaluation. This includes an oro facial examination, 'dry swallows', and, based on these findings, trial swallows with appropriate amounts and consistencies. At the bedside it is not possible to identify, with 100% certainty, if aspiration is occurring or not. If it is suspected, a radiographic evaluation is the ideal diagnostic procedure. The modified barium swallow/videofluoroscopy will:

- identify oropharyngeal symptoms, such as penetration, residue, and backflow;
- identify underlying anatomical and physiological deficits that are causing the symptoms;
- provide baseline measure of swallow functions;
- help determine strategies and consistencies that maximize the swallow efficiency and minimize the aspiration risk.

Possible screening procedures include: FEES (flexible fiberoptic endoscopy of swallowing), where the pharynx and larynx can be visualized before and after a swallow; and cervical auscultation, where the sound of swallowing in relation to respiration can aid in diagnosis.[31] These may be useful for reviewing and monitoring swallow function. Once assessment is completed, the findings can be discussed with the patient, relatives, and other members of the team, so that an appropriate management strategy can be planned.

Intervention in dysphagia

The speech and language therapist has many components to their role, apart from assessing dysphagia. For example:

- education about the swallowing process and assessment findings;
- indirect therapy, e.g. range of motion exercises to strengthen/maintain muscle movements;
- direct therapy, e.g. thermal, tactile stimulation to improve efficiency of the trigger of the pharyngeal swallow;
- teach compensatory strategies:
  - postural changes, such as chin down—helpful when the pharyngeal swallow is delayed, as it widens the valleculae and narrows the airway entrance;
  - physical manoeuvres, such as the supraglottic swallow—helpful when there is a delayed pharyngeal swallow; reduced or late vocal cord closure, as voluntary breath hold usually closes the vocal cords before and during the swallow;[4]
- modify/change external variables, such as bolus size, consistency (e.g. thickened fluids for a delayed pharyngeal swallow), and temperature;
- regularly update and consult with the multi-professional team;
- assist with optimizing nutrition and hydration in the face of declining health.

Timing of intervention is important, as inevitably there will be a need for ongoing review of clinical decisions. Ideally, this requires the establishment and maintenance of an accessible, open, robust, and reliable communication system, amongst and between the hospital and community teams, and, of paramount importance, with the patient and their carers.

Early referral facilitates the development of rapport, trust, and shared knowledge with the patient and carers. Their perceptions and role are vital for appropriate clinical management. Early intervention alongside an open inclusive communication network can ease decision-making, especially in stressful, difficult circumstances. For example:

- discussing potential treatment side-effects, such as mucositis, candida, oral hygiene, fatigue, steroids, anti-emetics, taste changes;
- discussing contentious issues such as feeding and hydrating the patient who has a very short prognosis and is deteriorating daily;
- providing accurate, updated information;
- identifying limitations and providing the opportunity for changes of opinion;
- being the patients advocate.

If the dysphagia persists, recurs, or worsens, there is a constant shift of emphasis, ensuring that the intervention and management decisions remain appropriate.

The speech and language therapist needs to be competent and confident when differentiating where her/his role ends and the need for further specialized support begins. Their role in 'end stage' care with this dysphagic patient group is in sharp contrast to the acute neurological rehabilitation upon which their dysphagia training is based.[32]

End-of-life issues

Much has been written on the importance of team working within palliative care. Witnessing patients grappling with end-of-life issues may distress the healthcare professionals involved. It is a deeply personal, complex issue that is difficult to comprehend. Perhaps by giving some thought to our own mortality, and any preconceptions, will help the team to support each other, as well as the patient and their families. Neuberger[33] states that one of her main reasons for writing her book *Dying well* was the medical profession's general reluctance to discuss death, unless in a particular specialist context. Her book is a thought-provoking exploration of belief systems surrounding death, dying, and bereavement. It is not an area that is covered in detail within the speech and language therapy training. Gallaghher-Allred[34] writes about end-of-life issues and the dying process for both children and adults. It is written from a dietician's perspective but describes professional issues applicable to all the multi-professional team. Stanier[32] highlights five steps to better practice in end-of-life care:

(1) put patients, their families, and their changing needs and wishes first;

(2) be sensitive to beginnings, shifts, endings, and their implications;

(3) minimize symptons and risks, maximize quality and constantly monitor/review;

(4) ensure multidisciplinary working, preferably through an integrated care pathway;[35]

(5) recognize that support at the end-of-life is valuable to perceived quality of care.

This subject is discussed in more detail in Chapter 9.

Dysphagia case history: Peter

Medical history and treatment Peter, 65, was diagnosed with an aggressive menigioma of the right sphenoid wing. The tumour impinged onto the brain-stem and encased major arteries and cranial nerves. He presented with a 6-month history of dysaesthesia of the right face, scalp, and tongue, and with very occasional coughing with drinks, but, surprisingly, was otherwise asymptomatic. Peter received stereotactic radiotherapy treatment and his post-treatment complications included steroid-induced diabetes, peripheral neuropathy, raised intra-cranial pressure, cardiac arrest following an hypoxic episode when food was aspirated, cognitive changes with short term memory impairment.

Speech and language therapy intervention Peter was referred to SLT prior to his radiotherapy. He was an extrovert man who described eating and drinking as being one of his key pleasures and admitted that he would find it very difficult to accept and adjust to any changes with this aspect of his life. Videofluoroscopy indicated mildly reduced oral control but no signs of penetration or aspiration. He was monitored during the 6-week radiotherapy treatment and managed a normal diet. An overview of the swallowing process, dysphagia information, and management were discussed with Peter and his wife. Written guidelines for safe feeding management were given and they were encouraged to contact the department if there were any concerns regarding communication and/or swallowing problems. Four months later, Peter was re-referred following admission to the hospital's critical care unit (CCU), where pieces of unchewed meat were removed from his trachea. He was unable to tolerate another videofluoroscopy but a bedside evaluation revealed fluctuating oro-pharyngeal dysphagia with a delayed trigger of the pharyngeal swallow and reduced laryngeal elevation. He was at risk of aspirating oral intake but swallow rehabilitation was compromised by his cognitive impairment. His short-term memory and attention span were reduced, and there were periods of confusion. Peter was unable to tolerate a naso-gastric tube or direct swallow therapy so, to reduce the risk of aspiration, all feeding had to be supervised. The dieticians were concerned about his nutrition and hydration, their management being further complicated by his steroid-induced diabetes. Issues relating to Peter's feeding management necessitated daily meetings between the dietician, nursing staff, speech and language therapist, and family. To facilitate a consistent management approach, compensatory strategies were discussed with the hospital team and his family, and a written version left in his room. These included positioning, appropriate food consistencies, amount, and rate of feeding. Much time was spent with the family, as they found it extremely distressing to feed him. Peter was unable to recall the cause of his recent admission, nor understand the need for such a controlled and controlling approach to his eating and drinking. He continued to deteriorate and, after meeting with the medical team, the family was able to discuss end-of-life issues and state their wish to look after him at home. Peter was discharged home with full community support, where he died 2-weeks later. His wife contacted the speech and language therapist 2 months after Peter's death. She reported feeling very uncomfortable with how she had managed the situation in the time between the completion of the radiotherapy and Peter's admission to CCU. Her issue involved managing the difficult balance between respecting personal choices and Peter's deteriorating function. Peter had experienced increasing problems with swallowing but forbade her to mention this to anyone. His family had chosen to respect and collude with his decision. During the initial SLT assessment, Peter had clearly indicated that he was unlikely to admit to any future swallowing problems. His wife was able to acknowledge that she had respected her husband's wishes and, in the final weeks, had gained comfort knowing the risk of his choking was minimized. She reported this had given her and her family precious time to focus on the imminent loss of a loved husband, father, and friend.

Summary

This chapter has touched on the very real professional and personal challenges for the speech and language therapist working with people diagnosed with primary brain tumours. It is not surprising that there is a paucity of good quality research for the management and therapy treatment for the acquired communication problems. Frequently the patients are not only facing a limited prognosis, but also experience fluctuating clinical presentations. This means that rigorous, formal testing can feel inappropriate and demoralizing. The results may emphasize all the things they *cannot* do.

To move forward, good qualitative and quantitative research is essential. An example of a potential contributor to this is the current development of an assessment where the focus is not on the impairment but on the impact of living with aphasia.[36] Rather than avoid the 'grey' areas of emotions, it provides an opportunity for the person with aphasia to reflect on areas relevant to their own lives. The sense, and impact, of losing their identity can easily be overlooked, especially when their world is suddenly governed by their medical diagnosis, prognosis, ongoing treatments, and side-effects. With this assessment, the whole person is acknowledged and their perceptions elicited, shared, and respected. Aspirations for us all, not just the people diagnosed with a primary brain tumour.

References

1 Lindsay, K. W. and Bone, I. (1997). *Neurology and neurosurgery illustrated* (3rd edn). Edinburgh: Churchill Livingstone.

2 Darley, F., Aronson, A., and Brown, J. (1975). *Motor speech disorders.* London: W. B. Saunders.

3 Duffy, J. E. (1995). *Motor speech disorders. Substrates, differential diagnosis and management.* St. Louis: Mosby, Inc.

4 Logemann, J. A. (1998). *Evaluation and treatment of swallowing disorders* (2nd edn). Texas: Pro-Ed Inc.

5 Murdoch, B. E. (1999). *Communication disorders in childhood cancers.* London: Whurr Publishers.

6 Murdoch, B. E. (1990). *Acquired speech and language disorders. A neuro-anatomical and functional neurological approach.* London: Chapman and Hall.

7 Sullivan, P. and Guilford, A. M. (ed.). (1999). *Swallowing intervention in oncology.* San Diego: Singular Publishing Group Inc.

8 Pound, C., Parr, S., Lindsay, J. *et al.* (2000). *Beyond aphasia, therapies for living with communication disability.* Oxon: Winslow Press Ltd.

9 Frank, A. W. (1995). *The wounded storyteller.* Chicago: Chicago University Press.

10 Greenhalgh, T. and Hurwitz, B. (ed.) (1999). *Narrative based medicine.* London: BMJ Books.

11 Fisher, S. (1998). Multidisciplinary teamwork. In *Neuro-oncology for nurses* (ed. D. Guerrero), pp.221–52. London: Whurr Publishers.

12 Embling, S. (1995). Exploring multidisciplinary teamwork. *Br J Ther Rehab* 2 (3), 142–4.

13 Lynch, B. L. (1981). Team building: will it work in health care? *J All Health* (November), 241.

14 Robinson, S. N. (1992a). The family with cancer. *Eur J Cancer Care* 1 (2), 29–33.

15 Robinson, S. N. (1992b). The learning needs of cancer patients. *Eur J Cancer Care* 1 (3), 18–20.

16 Caplan, D. (1987). *Neurolinguistic and linguistic aphasiology: an introduction.* Cambridge: Cambridge University Press.

17 Jacobs, D. H. (2002). Aphasia. *eMedicine Journal,* 3 (2), 1–13. *www.emedicine.com/neuro/topic437.htm.*

18 Gaziano, J. E. and Kumar, R. (1999). Primary brain tumours. In *Swallowing intervention in oncology* (ed. P. Sullivan and A. M. Guilford), pp.65–76. San Diego: Singular Publishing Group, Inc.

19 Scheibal, R. S., Meyers, C. A., and Levin, V. A. (1996). Cognitive dysfunction following surgery for intra-cerebral glioma. Influence of histopathology, lesion, location and treatment. *J Neuro-oncol* **30**, 61–9.

20 Kibler, S. (1998). Psychological support. In *Neuro-oncology for nurses* (ed. D. Guerrero), pp.271–93. London: Whurr Publishers.

21 Parr, S., Byng, S., Gilpin, S. and Ireland, C. (1997). *Talking about aphasia.* Buckingham: Open University Press.

22 Guerrero, D. (1998). In *Neuro-oncology for nurses* (ed. D. Guerrero), pp.151–77. London: Whurr Publishers.

23 Kagan, A. (1995). Revealing the competence of aphasic adults through conversation: a challenge to health care professionals. *Topics Stroke Rehab* **2** (1), 15–28.

24 Kagan, A. (1998). Supported conversation for adults with aphasia: methods and resources for training conversation partners. *Aphasiology* **12** (9), 816–30.

25 Kagan, A., Winckel, J., and Schumway, E. (1996). *Pictographic communication resources manual.* North York, Toronto: Aphasia Centre.

26 Le Dorze, G. and Brassard, C. (1995). A description of the consequences of aphasia on aphasic persons and their relatives and friends: based on the WHO model of chronic diseases. *Aphasiology* **9** (3), 239–56.

27 Parr, S. (1995). Everyday reading and writing in aphasia; role change and the influence of pre-morbid literary practice. *Aphasiology* **9** (3), 223–38.

28 Salter, M. (1998). Altered body image. In *Neuro-oncology for nurses* (ed. D. Guerrero), pp.151–77. London: Whurr Publishers.

29 Regnard, C. F. B. (1987). Dysphagia. *Balliere's Clinical Oncology* **1** (2), 327–55.

30 Bleach, N. R. (1993). The gag reflex and aspiration: a retrospective analysis of 120 patients assessed by videofluoroscopy. *Clinical Otolaryngeal* **18**, 303–7.

31 Zenner, P. M., Losinski, D. S., and Mills, R. H. (1995). Using cervical auscultation in the clinical dysphagia examination in long-term care. *Dysphagia* **10**, 27–31.

32 Stanier, J. (2002). A shift of emphasis. *Speech Lang Ther Pract* Autumn, 8–11.

33 Neuberger, J. (1999). *Dying well. A guide to enabling a good death.* Cheshire: Hochland and Hochland Ltd.

34 Gallagher-Allred, C. R. (1989). *Nutritional care of the terminally ill.* Maryland: Aspen Publishers Inc.

35 Ellershaw, J., Foster, A., Murphy, D. *et al.* (1997). Developing an integrated pathway for the dying patient. *Eur J Pall Care* **4**, 203–7.

36 Swinburn, K. and Byng, S. (2003). *Personal communication.* London: Connect.

Chapter 8

Nutritional problems in patients with primary cerebral malignancies

Mohammad Z. Al-Shahri and
Robin L. Fainsinger

Introduction

Food and feeding is crucial for maintaining life for all living creatures. In the human culture, food is central, not only for maintaining life but also for the way of living. Feeding has physical, psychosocial, and spiritual dimensions in life, and disturbances in nutritional status are likely to have significant implications. There is minimal literature about nutritional problems in patients with primary cerebral malignancies. The information discussed in this chapter concerning primary cerebral tumours will be based on the authors' clinical experience, in addition to the scarce published material on the subject. The majority of references listed at the end of this chapter are non-specific and pertain to cancer-related nutritional problems in general. The discussion covers, in general terms, the assessment of nutritional problems and gives an outline of a management plan. Dysphagia is discussed specifically in Chapter 7.

Causes of nutritional disturbances

Nutritional problems are remarkably high among cancer patients, with cachexia being manifested by approximately 80% of patients.[1] Nutritional problems in patients with primary cerebral malignancies could be caused by various pathophysiological mechanisms (Table 8.1). Responsible aetiologies in the individual patient are usually multi-factorial, rather than attributable to one isolated mechanism. Careful assessment is usually the foundation for a successful management plan.

Table 8.1 Causes of nutritional problems in patients with primary cerebral malignancies

- Cancer anorexia cachexia syndrome
- Impaired cognition
- Xerostomia
- Nausea and vomiting
- Psychological disturbances
- Smell and taste disturbances
- Dysphagia
- Cancer treatment complications

Impaired cognition

Patients with primary cerebral malignancies are prone to the development of cognitive impairment relatively early in the course of their disease. The difficulty in maintaining adequate nutritional intake is among the main problems for those with impaired cognition.

Nausea and vomiting

In addition to the emetogenic effect of the malignancy and some of its treatments, brain tumours are likely to cause more nausea and vomiting due to the pressure effect of the tumour and increased intra-cranial pressure.

Psychological disturbances

Cancer patients with untreated depression often lose interest in pleasurable activities such as food intake.

Complications of cancer treatment

Chemotherapy and radiation treatment can precipitate nutritional impairment by inducing nausea, vomiting, mucositis, and xerostomia.

Cachexia

This prevalent cancer manifestation is characterized by significant weight loss (more than 10% of pre-morbid weight) associated with loss of muscle mass, body fat, and visceral protein. Although cachexia is not necessarily correlated with tumour stage or burden, it has been associated with reduced survival.[2]

Thought once to be merely due to decreased oral intake, cancer cachexia is now believed to be a complex syndrome involving tumour–host interactions leading to specific alterations in carbohydrate, protein, and lipid metabolism.[1] The symptom complexes associated with cachexia include anorexia, chronic nausea, early satiety, asthenia, and changes in body image. In our clinical experience, the cachexia syndrome is not a predominant or prevalent cause for nutritional problems in primary cerebral malignancies.

Anorexia

Anorexia implies the subjective feeling of loss of appetite and the consequent hypophagia. The aetiology in cancer patients involves the interplay between psychogenic, tumour-related, and treatment-induced factors.[1] Mucositis, nausea/vomiting, and disturbances in taste and smell can contribute to anorexia. Tumour–host interactions mediated by cytokines are also believed to play a detrimental role on appetite. Another possible cause for loss of appetite in brain tumour patients is impaired cognition.

Taste and smell abnormalities

Alterations in taste and smell are known to be associated with cancer. Food may have a metallic or a cotton-wool taste for some patients receiving chemotherapy.[3] Another observation is the heightened sense of olfaction and bitter taste noted by some cancer patients.[4] Inferior frontal-lobe tumours involving central olfactory pathways could lead to disturbances in olfaction. Generally, patients do not spontaneously complain of alterations in taste or smell, but rather need to be asked what specifically made them avoid certain foods.

Xerostomia

Xerostomia or dry mouth is one of the common symptoms among cancer patients. Dry mouth in cancer patients could be precipitated by cancer treatment, medications (especially opioids and anticholinergics), dehydration, psychological distress, and oral infections.

Dysphagia

Difficulty in transferring solids or liquids from the mouth to the stomach is found in more than one-tenth of cancer patients in general.[5] Patients with brain tumours could suffer impairment of oral intake simply because of impaired cognition. Disturbed swallowing mechanism could also occur due to tumours involving the swallowing centre, located in the pons and medulla oblongata. Other causes of dysphagia are not specific to brain tumours and include xerostomia, infection, and psychological distress.

Assessment

Careful evaluation of the possible causes of nutritional problems in the individual patient is the first step towards a specifically tailored management plan. The fact that cancer is the ultimate culprit in causing the problem should not preclude looking for potentially correctable or modifiable contributory factors. Evaluation of the extent of the problem is as important.

General assessment

The patient's general condition should be assessed in terms of performance status, prognosis, and expected longevity. The meaning of the nutritional problem and its impact on the patient and family from their own perspective should also be explored.

Specific assessments

Appetite

This could be assessed using a visual analogue or a numerical scale as is the case in the Edmonton Symptom Assessment Scale (ESAS).[6] Otherwise, simple description of appetite by the patient or caregiver as 'good', 'fair', or 'poor' may suffice for initial assessment and follow-up evaluations. In patients with far advanced disease and limited life-expectancy, frequent assessment of appetite is not warranted, as this symptom appears more stable over time compared to the common symptoms suffered by cancer patients approaching the end-stages of life.[7]

Caloric intake

Methods that aim at objectively assessing caloric intake are mainly employed for research purposes rather than day-to-day patient care. For the latter purpose, a reasonably reliable method is to have trained nurses estimate percentages of food portions consumed by patients.[8]

Body nutritional status

Various assessment methods are used to evaluate the nutritional status and body composition. Some of these are simple, such as anthropometric measurements, while others are moderately or highly sophisticated, such as infra-red interactance, dynamometry, absorptiometry, whole body potassium estimation, bioimpedance, and electroconductivity studies and radiologic imaging techniques. In palliative-care settings, given the limited life-expectancy of patients and the marginal possibility of reversing significant nutritional problems, sophisticated measures for assessing body nutritional status are not usually warranted. Assessment of body weight changes, serum levels of albumen, haemoglobin, magnesium, and electrolytes, all in the context of basic bedside clinical observation, could act as more practically useful indicators of the nutritional status.

Assessment of associated problems

The complex multi-dimensional nature of nutritional problems in patients with cerebral malignancies needs to be considered. Asthenia is a recognized symptom in the majority of cancer patients with advanced disease and thought to be in close association with cancer cachexia.[9] Psychological distress has also been reported to have clear association with cachexia.[10] On the one hand, patient and family might perceive decreased oral intake and progressive weight loss as signs of impending death. On the other hand, depression could lead to anorexia and consequent significant nutritional problems. The progressive physical decline, ascites, and lower limb oedema associated with the anorexia/asthenia/cachexia syndrome, is likely to result in physical discomfort and aggravate the complaints of pain.[11] Some reports suggest that cancer cachexia contributes to respiratory muscle weakness resulting in dyspnea.[12]

Management plan

Although the focus of this chapter is basically on a seemingly homogeneous group of cancer patients, i.e. those with primary brain malignancies, the management plan will need to be specifically tailored to individual patients' needs, expectations, and preferences. Family members should be involved sooner rather than later in the planning phase. The goals of management should be discussed with patients and families before suggesting any decisions, and should be revisited periodically during the course of management. It could be beneficial at times to explain to patients and families that theoretical evidence suggests that artificial nutritional support in patients with cerebral malignancies could possibly nourish the tumour and foster its growth more than benefiting the patient.[13-14] Generally, the effect of nourishment in patients with advanced cancer is not likely to have positive impact on survival or quality of life.[15-16] Management, therefore, should be mainly comfort-centred and designed to improve symptom control and heighten patients' sense of well-being. The patients' and families' concerns might be focused on such symptoms like impaired oral intake, nausea, body image changes, and asthenia.

An interdisciplinary approach should be adopted in the design and execution of a management plan. The patient's prognosis needs to be discussed with the oncologist, neurosurgeon, or radiation oncologist involved in the management of the case. Swallowing assessment could usually be arranged by an occupational therapist. The dietitian's role is vital in the assessment of nutritional status and dietary needs. Dietitians can also provide recommendations on various dietary options for the particular patient and also for modification of diets as the need arises along the course of the illness. Other team members could help to address psychosocial and spiritual issues, and significantly contribute to the success of the overall management plan.

General considerations

One of the possibly controllable causes of impaired nutritional intake in brain tumour patients is the increased intra-cranial pressure leading to nausea, vomiting, and disturbed cognition. This is often controlled by dexamethasone, which usually improves symptoms in less than 48 h. If the nutritional problem is caused mainly by xerostomia and mouth ulcers, proper mouth care, artificial saliva, and analgesics may lead to significant improvement. Clinically depressed patients need to be diagnosed and treated as early as possible.

The oral route is generally the preferred route for nutritional intake, as long as the patient's condition so permits. In patients with advanced cancer, enteral and parenteral nutrition is usually reserved for a limited number of patients, partly because of the side-effects and the discomfort associated with these routes, and also due to the limited potential for improving patients' well-being. However, a patient with impaired swallowing and a level of consciousness close to normal, with a life-expectancy of several weeks to few months, could benefit from an enteral feeding via a gastrostomy tube.

Pharmacological management

Corticosteroids

Dexamethasone in a dose of 4–8 mg daily, or an equivalent dose of prednisone, is believed to be associated with a few weeks improvement in appetite.[17] Corticosteroids are, therefore, a good choice for stimulating the appetite of patients with life-expectancy of days to a few weeks. Steroids may also have other favourable effects, such as control of nausea and improved sense of well-being. These effects of corticosteroids are postulated to be mediated by its central euphoriant activity and inhibition of cytokine activity, in addition to its effects on prostaglandin metabolism.[18–19] Dexamethasone in higher doses can sometimes dramatically improve cognition, and control nausea and vomiting in patients with increased intra-cranial pressure.

Metoclopramide

This anti-dopaminergic drug has a central anti-emetic effect, as well as a gastro-intestinal prokinetic effect, and, hence, its positive effects on nausea control and appetite stimulation in patients with advanced cancer who are often on opioids and prone to autonomic failure.[17] Due to the short half-life of this medication, some patients need more frequent administration or the use of controlled release formula, or even a continuous infusion, to achieve the desired effect.

Megestrol acetate

This progestational drug has shown some capability of reducing nausea, improving appetite, and increasing caloric intake in cancer patients with advanced disease.[20] Doses of 160–800 mg/day are likely to show beneficial effects in less than 2 weeks.[21] For cost-containment purposes, and to reduce the potential for dose-related side-effects, the recommended approach is to start with a low dose (160–480 mg/day) and gradually titrate upwards.

Other pharmacological options

Cannabinoids

Different cannabinoids (e.g. dronabinol and nabilone) have shown some appetite-stimulating effects.[17,22] The central side-effects, and the modest effect on cancer anorexia/cachexia syndrome, are among the reasons for limited use of these agents in patients with advanced cancer.[20,22]

Omega-3 fatty acids

Eicosapentanoic acid (EPA) is a major omega-3 fatty acid constituent of fish oil, which may induce weight gain in patients with cancer cachexia.[23] More controlled trials are needed to strengthen the current evidence on this agent.

Non-steroidal anti-inflammatory drugs (NSAIDs)

Some NSAIDs (e.g. ibuprofen) were found to contribute to significant weight gain in cancer patients.[24] This needs to be clarified further by well designed randomized controlled trials.

Thalidomide

The limited work on using this agent in human immunodeficiency virus (HIV) infected and cancer patients has shown promising effects on appetite and weight gain.[25] More studies are expected to evaluate the potential symptomatic benefits of this drug in patients with advanced cancer.

Melatonin

The limited evidence on this agent so far suggests potential beneficial effect on cancer cachexia, as well as on chemotherapy-induced fatigue.[26]

Hydrazine sulfate

Despite some promising initial reports, randomized controlled trials showed this agent to have no significant effect on appetite or weight in patients with advanced cancer.[27] However, the agent is still widely used by alternative therapists to treat anorexia/cachexia in cancer patients.

Cyproheptadine

This is an anti-serotoninregic agent with appetite-enhancing effects.[28] However, its effect on body weight is not as promising, and its sedative effect limits its usefulness in patients with cerebral malignancies.

Ethical considerations

The great importance given to nutrition is due to the fact that persistent starvation eventually ends in death. Following diagnosis with cancer, patients and families might look at good nutrition as one of the weapons that could help to 'beat' cancer. When the cancer grows beyond available curative measures and becomes far advanced, patients and their families may consider food intake as one of the few remaining enjoyable activities the patient can have. These factors emphasize the sensitivity of issues concerning nutrition in cancer population. The ethical considerations pertinent to nutritional problems in cancer population are many (Table 8.2).[29] Decisions on ethical issues should always be made by a group rather than an individual person. The patient, family, and health-team members should be involved. Ethical committees in a health institution are occasionally consulted. Before decisions are made, thorough assessment should include the patient's own priorities and clinical condition, symptoms, life-expectancy, hydration/nutritional status, spontaneous/voluntary nutritional intake, psychological status, and available options in terms of routes of administration.[30] Following an intervention, re-evaluation of the whole management process should be repeated at specific intervals.

Table 8.2 Ethical considerations concerning management of nutritional problems in advanced cancer patients

- Whether to intervene?
- Who decides? On what?
- When to reevaluate decisions?
- Withholding versus withdrawing?
- Definition of futility. Who should define it?
- Definition of 'terminal'.
- The role of 'uncertainty' regarding outcomes of withholding and withdrawing.
- Adults versus children.
- The role of religious beliefs.
- Professionals' beliefs and concerns
- Legal considerations

Assessment of outcomes

In clinical practice, interventions intended for managing nutritional problems in patients with advanced cancer are more likely to improve intake of nutrients, than to improve body weight and to restore body image. The desired outcomes of such interventions include improved sense of well-being, maintaining pleasure of eating, and enjoying the social benefits from sharing food with family and friends. These outcome measures were incorporated in the Bristol–Myers Anorexia Cachexia Recovery Instrument (BACRI), which was validated on patients with HIV-related wasting treated with megestrol acetate.[31]

Conclusions

Nutritional problems can have serious detrimental effects on the quality of life for patients with advanced cerebral malignancies. In addition to the possibility of cancer anorexia/cachexia syndrome, patients with cerebral malignancies are prone to intra-cranial tumour pressure effect leading to nausea/vomiting and disturbed level of consciousness with further deterioration in nutritional status. The recommended approach for management includes comprehensive assessment, and early involvement of the patient and family in making decisions and setting goals. An interdisciplinary team has a better chance of success in managing such complex and multi-factorial problems.

References

1 Strasser, F. and Bruera, E. (2002). Update on anorexia and cachexia. *Hematol Oncol Clin North Am* **16** (3), 589–617.

2 Davis, M. P. and Dickerson, D. (2000). Cachexia and anorexia: cancer's covert killer. *Support Care Cancer* **8** (3), 180–7.

3 Wickham, R. S., Rehwaldt, M., Kefer, C. *et al.* (1999). Taste changes experienced by patients receiving chemotherapy. *Oncol Nurs Forum* **26** (4), 697–706.

4 Ovesen, L., Sorensen, M., Hannibal, J. *et al.* (1991). Electrical taste detection thresholds and chemical smell detection thresholds in patients with cancer. *Cancer* **68** (10), 2260–5.

5 Sykes, N. P., Baines, M., and Carter, R. L. (1988). Clinical and pathological study of dysphagia conservatively managed in patients with advanced malignant disease. *Lancet* **2** (8613), 726–8.

6 Bruera, E., Kuehn, N., Miller, M. J. *et al.* (1991). The Edmonton Symptom Assessment System (ESAS), a simple method for the assessment of palliative care patients. *J Palliat Care* **7** (2), 6–9.

7 Dudgeon, D. J., Harlos, M., and Clinch, J. J. (1999). The Edmonton Symptom Assessment Scale (ESAS) as an audit tool. *J Palliat Care* **15** (3), 14–9.

8 Bruera, E., Chadwick, S., Cowan, L. *et al.* (1986). Caloric intake assessment in advanced cancer patients: comparison of three methods. *Cancer Treat Rep* **70** (8), 981–3.

9 Bruera, E. and MacDonald, R. N. (1988). Asthenia in patients with advanced cancer. Issues in symptom control. Part 1. *J Pain Symptom Manage* **3** (1), 9–14.

10 Higginson, I. and Winget, C. (1996). Psychological impact of cancer cachexia on the patient and family. In: *Cachexia-anorexia in cancer patients* (ed. E. Bruera and I. Higginson), pp.172–83. Oxford: Oxford University Press.

11 Gerber, L. H. (2001). Cancer rehabilitation into the future. *Cancer* **92** (Suppl. 4), 975–9.

12 Dudgeon, D. J., Lertzman, M., and Askew, G. R. (2001). Physiological changes and clinical correlations of dyspnea in cancer outpatients. *J Pain Symptom Manage* **21** (5), 373–9.

13 Munro, H. N. (1977). Tumour-host competition for nutrients in the cancer patient. *J Am Diet Assoc* **71** (4), 380–4.

14 Torosian, M. H. and Daly, J. M. (1986). Nutritional support in the cancer-bearing host. Effects on host and tumour. *Cancer* **58** (Suppl. 8), 1915–29.

15 Koretz, R. L. (1984). Parenteral nutrition: is it oncologically logical? *J Clin Oncol* **2** (5), 534–8.

16 Detsky, A. S., Baker, J. P., O'Rourke, K. *et al.* (1987). Perioperative parenteral nutrition: a meta-analysis. *Ann Intern Med* **107** (2), 195–203.

17 Nelson, K. A., Walsh, D., and Sheehan, F. A. (1994). The cancer anorexia-cachexia syndrome. *J Clin Oncol* **12** (1), 213–25.

18 Fainsinger, R. (1996). Pharmacological approach to cancer anorexia and cachexia. In: *Cachexia-anorexia in cancer patients* (ed. E. Bruera and I. Higginson), pp.128–40. Oxford: Oxford University Press.

19 Plata-Salaman, C. R. (1991). Dexamethasone inhibits food intake suppression induced by low doses of interleukin-1 beta administered intracerebrovntricularly. *Brain Res Bull* **27** (5), 737–8.

20 Jatoi, A., Windschitl, H. E., Loprinzi, C. L. *et al.* (2002). Dronabinol versus megestrol acetate versus combination therapy for cancer-associated anorexia: a North Central Cancer Treatment Group study. *J Clin Oncol* **20** (2), 567–73.

21 Bruera, E., Ernst, S., Hagen, N. *et al.* (1998). Effectiveness of megestrol acetate in patients with advanced cancer: a randomized, double-blind, crossover study. *Cancer Prev Control* **2** (2), 74–8.

22 Beal, J. E., Olson, R., Laubenstein, L. *et al.* (1995). Dronabinol as atreatment for anorexia associated with weight loss in patients with AIDS. *J Pain Symptom Manage* **10** (2), 89–97.

23 Wigmore, S. J., Barber, M. D., Ross, J. A. *et al.* (2000). Effect of oral eicosapentaenoic acid on weight loss in patients with pancreatic cancer. *Nutr Cancer* **36** (2), 177–84.

24 McMillan, D. C., Wigmore, S. J., Fearon, K. C. *et al.* (1999). A prospective randomized study of megestrol acetate and ibuprofen in gastrointestinal cancer patients with weight loss. *Br J Cancer* **79** (3–4), 495–500.

25 Inui, A. (2002). Cancer anorexia-cachexia syndrome: current issues in research and management. *CA Cancer J Clin* **52** (2), 72–91.

26 Lissoni, P. (2002). Is there a role for melatonin in supportive care? *Support Care Cancer* **10** (2), 110–6.

27 Loprinzi, C. L., Kuross, S. A., O'Fallon, J. R. *et al.* (1994). Randomized placebo-controlled evaluation of hydrazine sulfate in patients with advanced colorectal cancer. *J Clin Oncol* **12** (6), 1121–5.

28 Pawlowski, G. J. (1975). Cyproheptadine: weight-gain and appetite stimulation in essential anorexic adults. *Curr Ther Res Clin Exp* **18** (5), 673–8.

29 British Medical Association (2001). *Withholding and withdrawing life-prolonging medical treatment: guidance for decision making.* London: BMJ Books.

30 Bozzetti, F., Amadori, D., Bruera, E. *et al.* (1996). Guidelines on artificial nutrition versus hydration in terminal cancer patients. European Association for Palliative Care. *Nutrition* **12** (3), 163–7.

31 Cella, D. F., Von Roenn, J., Lloyd, S. *et al.* (1995). The Bristol-Myers Anorexia /Cachexia Recovery Instrument (BACRI), a brief assessment of patients' subjective response to treatment for anorexia/cachexia. *Qual Life Res* **4** (3), 221–31.

Chapter 9

The last days of life

Odette Spruyt

Care begins when difference is recognised[1]

Caring for the patient who is dying calls for both the clinical expertise and the humanity of the medical team. There is an urgency, power, and poignancy in accompanying people during their last days of life, which impacts on the usual boundaries of care. Cassem outlined the general duties of physicians at this time, many of which extend beyond the clinical domain.[2] Often it is the non-clinical aspects of end-of-life care that challenge the physician most.[3]

What is specific to end-of-life care for patients with primary and secondary brain tumours?

- Primary brain tumours commonly occur in younger patients, e.g. anaplastic astrocytomas, which account for 20–40% of high-grade astrocytomas, occur most commonly in patients between 30 and 50 years of age.[4]

- Mental status change may be an early and persistent feature, and aggravated by therapies such as whole-brain radiotherapy[5] or chemotherapy.

- Communication may be severely disturbed with dysphasia or dysarthria, delirium, and reduced level of consciousness making assessment, monitoring, and discussion of preferences for end-of-life care difficult.

- The patient's appearance may be greatly altered after weeks or months of steroids.

- Dying may be prolonged and time of death difficult to predict.

- Carers are often asked by health professionals to act as proxy reporters of symptoms and patients' wishes. Functional loss may be profound from presentation, with the resultant dependence on carers for assistance. This may be difficult to sustain throughout the illness and with increasing degrees of debility. The changes in roles and dynamics in relationships may also be profound, sudden, and early, with carers assuming new and additional responsibilities previously the domain of the patient. Secondary tumours to the brain are seldom solitary metastases. Therefore, morbidity from other sites of disease complicates management and at times, may dominate the clinical picture.

Box 9.1 Commonly encountered ethical issues in end-of-life care

The offering or withholding of parenteral nutrition or fluids.

The extent of intervention desired in possible future clinical scenarios, including ventilatory support and cardiopulmonary resuscitation.

The nature of symptom control and aggressive palliation in the event of intolerable distress in the last days of life.

The nomination of others as proxy decision-makers.

Interpreting the patient's wishes for care in changing clinical circumstances.

Place of death

Determining the patient's preferred place of death is a key aspect of individualizing care. For patients with brain tumors, early consideration and discussion of end-of-life care is important, as subsequent cognitive deterioration in the course of illness may preclude such discussions. The timing of such discussions with patient and family, i.e. 'those for whom the patient matters',[6] always calls for sensitive acknowledgement of the grief and distress associated with broaching such topics, as well as knowledge of the cultural and particular outlook of that patient/family group. It is worth noting that often in end-of-life care, discussion of practical issues, such as planning for preferred place of death, often leads on to discussion of ethical, prognostic, and other sensitive issues. Commonly encountered ethical issues are listed in Box 9.1.

Cause of death

In general, in the cancer patient population, unexpected death is uncommon, occurring in approximately 10–15% of all deaths. Causes of sudden death in patients with primary or secondary brain tumours include massive haemorrhage from cerebral tumour or other sites of metastatic spread, coning of the brainstem, infarction and secondary oedema within cerebral tumour, anoxia secondary to status epilepticus, overwhelming sepsis, e.g. chemotherapy/ radiotherapy complication, and complications of tumour at other sites, e.g. cardiac tamponade. Suicide is an uncommon cause of death in patients with all types of cancer. More commonly, death in patients with primary or secondary brain tumours is anticipated, with dying occurring over days to weeks. Care needs to be taken not to prolong suffering and dying with unwise interventions. Dialogue with the family and within the extended team is vital at all times to ensure clarity of intention and shared goals of care.

How to approach a patient who is comatose and dying

Doctors often feel very awkward when entering a room where the patient is unconscious and is surrounded by tired, anxious, and expectant family. The importance of such ongoing visits to family is worth stressing. Many questions and uncertainties arise in the hours of watching and being with patients, questions that may assume considerable intensity. It may be the sense of the lack of remedy, the lack of answers, which deters doctors from continuing contact at this time, for fear of experiencing helplessness and failure. Equipped with the acceptance of death, such encounters are less threatening. Despite the inability to alter the fact of imminent death, the doctor's presence and non-abandonment provides powerful reassurance to the family that all that can be done is being done, that death is not a result of lack of care or expertise. More positively, the doctor can address questions as they arise and before they become a source of conflict within the family or between the family and the caring team. The doctor can do much to encourage resolution of conflict within the family group and a sense of calm and order around the patient. At times, with large family groups, it is necessary to ask for only two or three representatives to remain during such reviews.

Daily examination of the patient should commence with bedside observation, assessing the general comfort of the patient, the colour of the trunk and extremities, respiratory pattern, level of consciousness, and the level of peacefulness or distress amongst the family members. Good comfort care includes the following nursing management—in many countries these tasks fall to the family to provide, and the role of the team is to teach and assist the family.

- Protection of pressure areas with use of air mattresses or other pressure area mattresses, application of emollients with gentle massage to maintain skin circulation, and frequent repositioning of limbs and posture until such movement becomes problematic for the patient.

- Airway protection with correct positioning on the side, encouraging deep breathing, and assisted coughing.

- Assistance with drinking and eating as fatigue and frailty increases. Often this is overlooked in a busy ward and there is an important role for family here. Supervision is needed at times to help family members feed safely and also to guide them in reducing the feeding as the patient weakens.

- Maintaining excellent oral hygiene with mouth swabs to moisten and cleanse the oral mucosa, mouthwashes and lubricants applied to the lips and oral mucosa. The family may also be encouraged to participate in this if they wish. A check of oral hygiene, including looking for the presence of hygiene swabs at the bedside, may lead to discussion with the family about maintenance of hydration and estimations of prognosis.

Bowel review and care requires daily vigilance. Gentle rectal examination may be needed to exclude impaction if the patient is restless and uncomfortable. Despite a small oral intake, constipation is a common problem at the end of life if active measures are not maintained. Urinary retention is an important cause of end-of-life restlessness. An indwelling catheter may also be indicated if the patient is unconscious or too weak to manage to walk or be taken to the toilet. Subcutaneous and other needle sites need vigilance as painful abscesses may develop rapidly.

Medication review

An important medical role is that of daily medication review. Frustration and distress for the patient and carers arise from failed efforts to diligently swallow prescribed medications. Discontinuing unnecessary oral medications before such distress arises, or changing from oral to subcutaneous or other parenteral routes, will enhance symptom control; for example, anti-hypertensives, oral hypoglycaemics, and cholesterol-lowering medications should be discontinued. Diuretics and other agents for the management of congestive heart failure may cause terminal delirium due to dehydration and may be discontinued in most patients. Symptom control may become less effective if unnecessary drugs are continued, as essential medication such as analgesics may be omitted in an attempt to reduce the number of drugs that the patient has to take. There may be ethical concerns surrounding stopping corticosteroids at the end of life. Often these are no longer contributing any useful benefit and may be stopped without weaning the dose. If signs of headache such as increased restlessness in the comatose patient occur as a result, a low subcutaneous dose can be continued. Any decision to cease such long-term therapy upon which the patient and family have come to rely and have experienced direct benefit during the course of their illness, must involve the patient and/or family.

In addition to actively stopping medications, it is important to ensure that emergency drugs such as parenteral opioids, sedatives, and anti-emetics are available. For most patients, a supply may safely be kept in the home for use in possible emergencies. End-of-life care involves anticipation of probable complications and active management of symptoms as they arise, with frequent review of medications and dosage/agent adjustment. This is an area where individualizing care, and preparing and skilling carers for such developments can make a great difference to the quality of dying.

Communication with the family

Once the patient is unconscious, interaction with the family becomes more directly focused on their needs. There is more opportunity for the family to talk about their own concerns about life after the death of the patient. Doctors often call upon other members of the team, such as pastoral care, social workers, and volunteers trained in bereavement care, to assist in the discussions and ongoing care, but should not overlook the important contribution they can make to effective grieving by sensitive interaction at this time. There now may be an opening for the doctor to check for risk factors such as lack of social support, substance abuse, history of depression, co-dependent or ambivalent relationship between patient and family member, or multiple bereavements. Young children and teenagers losing a parent often require specific assistance in bereavement, such as opportunities to farewell their parent in ways appropriate to their stage of development. Patients with brain tumours often undergo a 'piecemeal' death, and children may feel very distant to the dying parent by the time of actual death. Allowing expression of this distance, and helping the child to remember and stay in contact with their parent is an important task of caring teams.

Team work

Until recently, the limited options for active management for cerebral tumours meant that symptomatic management by the palliative care team was generally agreed by all members of the multidisciplinary teams involved, medical and radiation oncologists, neurosurgeons, and palliative-care providers. However, with developments in neurosurgery, stereotactic radiotherapy, and palliative chemotherapy, the decision-making has become more complex, raising the question 'which form of palliation?'. There is little data on survival and quality of life for each tumour type on which to base these decisions. It falls to clinical wisdom and individualized patient-centred care, to inform such decisions. Ideally there would be an opportunity for all disciplines to discuss the strategies available and come to an agreed plan of management, which can then be discussed with the patient and family. This requires close working relationships with all teams involved and opportunities for palliative care providers to influence decision-making. Hospital-based palliative-care teams are best placed to participate in such discussions and to provide insights into the broader aspects of management, such as the family needs and concerns. The question 'would you be surprised if (this patient/Mr/Ms N or your father, as appropriate) dies within the next 6 months?' has emerged as a useful trigger question to start addressing end-of-life issues with the patient, family, and teams involved.[7] As the imminence of death is increasingly recognized, a shift is required in management goals, in which the burden of any proposed 'palliative' management, including any further investigations, is increasingly weighted against the immediate and experienced benefit for the patient.

Specific issues in end-of-life care

Hydration

Commonly, concerns arise regarding fluid and food intake. Most families wish to take part in some aspects of physical care of the patient and, commonly, this domain of nutritional support remains accessible to them. They will usually need to be taught how to maintain moist mucous membranes and advised of the importance of this in reducing the discomfort of thirst.[8] Sensitive discussion of the cultural attitudes surrounding maintenance of fluid/food is necessary to achieve agreement. Professionals cannot expect this social domain of care to be handed over to them exclusively. Kanitsaki[9] writes of a family who persisted in offering hot broth and rice to their dying mother to counteract the cold water and ice being used by staff for oral hygiene. They believed this was unhealthy and weakening her further. They understood that she no longer needed nor could take food but felt obliged to 'balance' her temperature. Once the fluid for oral hygiene was warmed and the clear broth included as an oral hygiene liquid, they discontinued their attempts to feed her. Health professionals must be prepared to negotiate with the family and to make their recommendations to the family with humility.

The boundary between usual care and extraordinary care is blurred in this area. Most families can accept not offering enteral (nasogastric or percutaneous enterogastric) or parenteral forms of nutrition to the dying patient, with explanation of the intensive and uncomfortable nature of such management and its futility in this setting. However, more reassurance and explanation regarding fluids is needed. Subcutaneous infusion of fluids (hypodermoclysis) of 500–1000 ml/24 h avoids painful repeated intravenous cannulations and can be maintained at home. Clinical indications for hypodermoclysis include delirium secondary to dehydration and/or accumulation of opioid and other drug metabolic products.[10] At times, hypodermoclysis may be set up solely out of respect for the family's wishes.

This subject is also discussed in Chapter 8.

Symptom management

Good symptom management is a cornerstone of good end-of-life care. Common symptoms are listed in Box 9.2 and good reviews of management are contained in standard palliative care texts. The symptoms of pain, delirium, dyspnoea and terminal secretions will be discussed here.

Pain management

Pain continues to be experienced until deep unconsciousness ensues, so analgesics must be maintained throughout the course of the terminal phase, continuing previously effective analgesia as tolerated. Doses can be safely titrated by increments of 30–50% of the previous dose, until pain is relieved or side-effects necessitate an alternative approach. Once oral administration of analgesics is no longer possible, the parenteral route, preferably the subcutaneous route either via regular interval dosing or as a continuous infusion via a syringe driver or similar device, provides a simple alternative which is minimally invasive and able to be maintained in the home setting. Breakthrough medication at doses of 10–15% of the total 24-h dose is safe and effective

---

Box 9.2 Common symptoms/problems at the end-of-life in patients with primary or secondary brain tumours

Pain: headache—raised intracranial pressure; pain at other sites of disease

Dyspnoea

Delirium

Terminal secretions

Fatigue

Muscle ache

Convulsions

Nausea and vomiting

Steroids effects, e.g. hyperglycaemia, change in appearance (hirsutism, truncal obesity, striae, moon facies), infections (thrush, cellulitis) thrombophlebitis

for additional episodes of pain, which may occur. Stable analgesia can be considered to be a maintenance dose with less than three breakthrough doses in 24 h. However, incident pain occurring with movement remains a challenging area of pain management. The aim is to provide analgesia of short duration and rapid onset, without excessive increases in maintenance dose, which would result in opioid toxicity. For rapid relief, within 5 mins, an IV dose is most effective, in a dose equivalent of 20% total daily dose, remembering the route conversion calculation. In the example in Box 9.3, the dose would be 5 mg IV.

Editor's note: many units would use subcutaneous as first choice, unless there is an IV line in place.

Box 9.3 Case history, Mrs B: advanced carcinoma breast, cerebral metastases, cared for at home

Good analgesia with modified-release morphine 90 mg twice daily, orally.

Acute admission to cancer institute with sudden onset of severe nausea and vomiting, acute pain and terminal delirium. Oral medications discontinued, subcutaneous morphine commenced.

Modified-release morphine 90 mg twice daily = 180 mg morphine 24/h

3 : 1 conversion ratio, switching oral to subcutaneous route → 180 mg orally = 60 mg subcutaneous, commenced on morphine injection 10 mg q4h sc

Required three breakthrough doses of 10 mg over next 24 h, each within 30 min of next regular dose:

Total dose = 90 mg subcutaneous over 24 h (breakthrough + regular analgesia)

Dose titrated to morphine injection 15 mg q4h subcutaneous

One breakthrough dose (15 mg) over next 24 h, associated with movement

Good maintenance analgesia

Wished to go home for final day with family before admission to hospice: converted to continuous infusion via a syringe driver

morphine tartrate 90 mg/24h

breakthrough dose 15 mg prn (hourly as needed, to a maximum of 3 doses) to be administered by husband

Editor's note: some authorities use a conversion ratio of 2:1 for oral to s.c. morphine (3:1 for oral to i.v.).

Table 9.1 Opioid analgesics commonly used in end-of-life care and their relative potency, not recommended doses

Opioid	Parenteral (intra-muscular/ subcutaneous)	Oral	Half-life (h)	Comment
Morphine	10	30	2–4	Reduce dose and do not use fixed dose regimens in renal impairment/failure (Cr > 250).
Oxycodone	15	30	3–4	Lower incidence of hallucinations.
Hydromorphone	1.5	7.5	2–3	Less cognitive impairment in elderly/patients with renal failure. High potency and solubility useful for syringe drivers when large opioid doses required.
Methadone	10	20–30	15–120	Although average half-life of 24 h, dosing interval generally 4–8 h, therefore risk of accumulation when drug is initiated or increased. Not recommended in cognitively impaired.
Diamorphine	5	20–30	0.05	Rapidly biotransformed to morphine and acetyl morphine.
Fentanyl	0.1	Not applicable	1–2	Empirically, transdermal fentanyl 100 µg/h = 2–4 mg/h IV morphine. Not used IV in palliative care as potent respiratory depressant.

Selected commonly used opioid analgesics are listed in Table 9.1. Doses should always be titrated to suit individual patient requirements and response. The conversion factors given are a guide and cannot accurately predict for individual patient variation and cross-tolerance between opioids. Often the equi-analgesic doses calculated from such tables must be reduced significantly at times by as much as 75% or more of the calculated dose. While such opioid rotations are generally uncommon in the imminently dying patient, the emphasis on opioid side-effects as a cause of terminal delirium may result in an increasing tendency to change opioids in such patients and practitioners need to be aware of the pitfalls. In general, when dealing with complex pain problems, it is best to seek the advice of pain and palliative care specialists.

Transdermal analgesia may be maintained until death. It is inadvisable to commence the transdermal route in the imminently dying patient. The delayed time to therapeutic plasma levels, and lack of same drug breakthrough formulation in many countries, makes this a poor choice at this time. A syringe driver may be set up to deliver extra analgesia (e.g. morphine) but 'as needed' opioid doses for breakthrough pain should reflect the combined transdermal and subcutaneous dose. Intravenous administration is suitable, provided access is permanent, e.g. a porta Cath, thus avoiding multiple cannulations.

There is considerable confusion regarding the need for opioids in the terminal phase. Diagnosis of active dying does not automatically require the commencement of an opioid, contrary to common practice, and opioid doses used in the imminently dying in palliative-care units are often moderate, e.g. mean MEDD (Morphine Equivalent Daily Dose) increased from 42 mg to 55.5 mg parenterally.[11,12] Opioid side-effects can be distressing and severe, and are more common when used inappropriately, such as for sedation or when administered in excessive doses to hasten death. Conversely, opioids should be used actively, titrated rapidly to relieve pain according to guidelines,[13,14] and tailored to the individual.

Delirium

Delirium is common in patients with brain tumours and is one of the most distressing symptoms experienced by the patient and family. It may be either hyperactive delirium, where the patient is hyperalert, restless, agitated, with hallucinations, delusions, and hyperarousal (e.g. alcohol withdrawal syndrome), or hypoactive delirium, where the patient is hypoalert, lethargic, drowsy, and withdrawn (e.g. hepatic encephalopathy). Hypoactive delirium is commonly undetected, as the patient appears quiet and calm. However, it is distressing to the patient and it responds to therapy with anti-psychotic medications. Delirium calls for early diagnosis and aggressive management, which includes discontinuing all unnecessary medications, correcting dehydration if appropriate, ensuring patient safety (e.g. minimizing risk of falls, burns, and other accidents) and treatment with neuroleptics, aiming for early and effective control.[15] Physical restraint is not advised, but one-to-one nursing and watchfulness by staff or family members is often needed when delirium is most acute. The reassurance of familiar voices and faces can reduce the severity of the problem.

Dyspnoea

Dyspnoea is experienced by up to 80% of patients in the final week of life. Symptomatic benefit may be derived from opioids, bronchodilators, corticosteroids, mucolytics (including nebulized saline), and anxiolytics in addition to basic measures of correct positioning, and protection of airways and oxygen on an 'as-required' basis for symptomatic relief. Opioids, either continuously or intermittently administered, depending on the nature of the dyspnoea, provide effective relief by several mechanisms. The dose of opioid must be consistent with the current opioid dosage used for analgesia. In general, 15–20% of the 24-h dose will be effective, but individual dose finding will be necessary. In the opioid naïve patient, 1–5 mg orally (1–3 mg parenterally) q4h, depending on age, frailty, previous opioid history, renal function, and ability to supervise therapy, would be a safe starting dose. When dyspnoea is severe and the patient is imminently dying, deep sedation with benzodiazepines, neuroleptics such as chlorpromazine, methotrimeprazine, or olanzepine, or barbiturates may be indicated for optimum relief of distress.

Terminal secretions

Terminal secretions are a common manifestation in dying patients and the consequent noisy respirations may be very distressing to family members in attendance. Anti-muscarinic agents (see Box 9.4) are used to reduce type I (upper airway) secretions and may need to be given repeatedly. Tachyphylaxis appears to develop rapidly and may be overcome by titration of the dose to the desired effect. Anticholinergics, in particular atropine and hyoscine hydro-bromide, which cross the blood–brain barrier, may cause or aggravate agitated terminal delirium. Hyoscine butylbromide does not. Type II (lower airway) secretions are more likely to be infective. They may be copious and malodor-ous, and are more likely to develop when dying is prolonged. Single-dose, broad-spectrum antibiotics may relieve the volume and offensiveness of these secretions and should be considered, even in the pre-terminal phase, if their

Box 9.4 Drugs used for management of terminal secretions

Hyoscine hydrobromide 0.4 mg subcutaneous every 1–4 hours as needed; 0.8–3.2 mg/24 h subcutaneous continuous infusion

Glycopyrrolate 0.2–0.4 mg subcutaneous bolus then 0.6–1.2 mg/24 h subcutaneous continuous infusion

Atropine 0.6–1.2 mg subcutaneous every 4 hours

Hyoscine butyl bromide 20 mg subcutaneous q4h; 40–240 mg/24 h subcutaneous infusion

Broad spectrum antibiotics, e.g. ceftriaxone 1 gm intra-muscular immediately use would improve the quality of the carers' experience of accompanying the dying patient.[16] An uncommon cause of terminal secretions is neurogenic pulmonary oedema,[17] arising with abruptly increasing intracranial pressure.

Sedation in the imminently dying

Sedatives are frequently needed in end-of-life care for symptomatic relief of anxiety, dyspnoea, and agitation and insomnia. In most countries, the most commonly used sedatives are the benzodiazepines with midazolam the most frequently used agent and doses usually below 40 mg/24 h. However, the use of sedatives with the intention of producing deep sedation, so-called sedation of the imminently dying, ranges from 15 to 36% of patients, in international palliative-care practice. Delirium is the most common indication reported.[18] Neuroleptics, e.g. haloperidol or olanzepine, are the optimal choice for management of delirium, as benzodiazepines may aggravate it. However, if rapid, short-duration sedation is required, benzodiazepines are effective and widely available. Controversy has arisen over the use of sedatives, with some claiming that this is a surrogate form of euthanasia.[19,20] Keystones to good practice include early consultation when symptom management proves difficult, open discussion with patient/family and team about goals of care and available methods of achieving relief, documentation of management plans, clear charting of drugs and parameters for dose titration.[21] It is vital to achieve relief of severe distress and so use the means available intelligently and without fear. If physicians practice without duplicity, and respect the boundaries between relief of suffering and deliberate hastening of life, professional integrity will be maintained.

Crisis management

Despite the best planning and supportive care, crises still occur. Optimal management requires clarity of goals of care at that time. For example, if hyperactive terminal delirium from extensive cerebral leptomeningeal disease is recognized at an early stage of development, discussion of future deep sedation with the patient or, if they are no longer cognitively aware, with the family, would allow clinicians to control symptoms comprehensively with benzodiazepines or, if ineffective, with barbiturates. Phenobarbitone may be given by subcutaneous infusion and titrated to effective dose, usually in the range of 300–2400 mg/24 h. A loading dose of 100–300 mg slow IV may be required for rapid control. Tolerance may develop and results in frequent increments in dose. Barbiturates may cause hypersensitivity to pain and, in some patients, agitation rather than sedation. Box 9.5 provides suggestions for suitable medications and doses to use in such crises.

Box 9.5 Possible medications for use in crisis management

Midazolam: 5–10 mg subcutaneously

Diazepam: 5–10 mg p.r.

Chlorpromazine: 25–100 mg deep intra-muscular injection

Phenobarbitone: 100mg subcutaneously/intra-muscularly

Clonazepam: 2 mg sub-lingually/subcutaneously

Methotrimeprazine: 6.25–12.5 mg subcutaneously/intra-muscularly

– all agents should be repeated until the desired effect has been reached.

Clinical examples:

1 Patient on TTS fentanyl 100 μg/h
Morphine Equivalent Daily Dose (MEDD = 240–400 mg)

For emergency, morphine dose 20–40 mg

2 Patient on diazepam 10 mg daily for chronic anxiolysis
For emergency sedation in event of sudden crisis, e.g. haemorrhage, 10 mg diazepam injection, injectable preparation 1M, or midazolam 10 mg subcutaneously, and repeat as needed.

If suspect benzodiazepine tolerance: phenobarbitone 100–200 mg subcutaneously or chlorpromazine 50–100 mg deep intra-muscularly.

Other dimensions of care

The focus in this chapter has been on the more medical aspects of end-of-life care, as these are not well addressed in general medical and oncology texts. This is not to undermine the importance of the psycho-social dimensions, which are crucial to good care of the dying patient. To address these areas of care in the acute hospital setting can be very challenging, given the bustle of the environment, the lack of space, and the orientation toward more acute therapies and interventions. The recognition of the inevitability of death is a crucial aspect from which effective preparation for the end-of-life can occur. Assisting in this recognition is an important function of the palliative-care team. Those most closely involved with the patient may not recognize the signs of impending death as clearly. Families may also unburden their fears and doubts about survival and prognosis more readily to a team not involved in curative management, with less fear of disappointing the doctors and nurses who have worked with them over the preceding months in attempting to prolong life and achieve cure. Encouraging such discussions to surface allows planning and preparation for end-of-life to occur. Practical matters (financial arrangements, funeral plans, and specific issues around the future care of children) may need urgent attention. Reconciliations may need to occur, specific religious and spiritual duties may assume great urgency, outweighing the previous importance given to life-prolonging therapy, which demanded all the energy and attention of the patient and family. Supportive relationships, which will carry over into bereavement, may need to be established and nurtured. For many patients, a therapeutic crossroad is reached. Choices should be made with the best information and understanding of what is being chosen, so that the manner in which death occurs, despite its grief and sorrow, is nevertheless accompanied by a sense of peace arising out of some control and preparedness.

References

1　Frank, A. (2002). *At the will of the body: reflections on illness.* Boston: Houghton Mifflin.

2　Cassem, N. H. (1997). The dying patient In *Massachusetts General Hospital—handbook of general hospital psychiatry* (4th edn) (ed. N. H. Cassem, T. A. Stern, J. F. Rosenbaum *et al.*), pp.605–36. St Louis, Mosby-Year Book Inc.

3　Roy, D. (1995). Ethics and complexity in palliative care. *J Palliat Care* **11** (4), 3–4.

4　Laws, E. and Thapar, K. (1993). Brain tumours. *CA Cancer J Clin* **43**, 263–71.

5　Bezjak, A., Adam, J., Barton, R. *et al.* (2002). Symptom response after palliative radiotherapy for patients with brain metastases. *Eur J Cancer* **38** (4), 487–96.

6　Byock, I. R. (1996). The nature of suffering and the nature of opportunity at the end-of-life. *Clin Geriatr Med* **12** (2), 237–52.

7　Lynn, J. (2000). Finding the key to reform in end-of-life care. *J Pain Symptom Manage* **19** (3), 168–73.

8　Musgrave, C. F., Bartal, N., and Opstad, J. (1995). The sensation of thirst in dying patients receiving IV hydration. *J Palliat Care* **11** (4), 17.

9　Kanitsaki, O. (2002). Dying, death and grief *Nursing Review* June.

10　Bruera, E., Legris, M. A., Kuehn, N. *et al.* (1990). Hypodermoclysis for the administration of fluids and narcotic analgesics in patients with advanced cancer. *J Pain Symptom Manage* **5** (4), 218–20.

11　Portenoy, R. K. (1996). Morphine infusions at the end-of-life: the pitfalls in reasoning from anecdote. *J Palliat Care* **12** (4), 44–6.

12　Thorns, A. and Sykes, N. (2000). Opioid use in last week of life and implications for end-of-life decision-making. *Lancet* **356**, 398–9.

13　Expert working group of the research network of the European association for palliative care (2001). Morphine and alternative opioids in cancer pain: the EAPC recommendations. *British Journal of Cancer* **84** (5), 587–93.

14　Carver, A. and Foley, K. M. (2001). Symptom assessment and management. In *Neurology Clinics* (ed. A. Carver and K. M. Foley), pp.921–47.

15 Gagnon, P., Allard, P., Masse, B. *et al.* (2000). Delirium in terminal cancer a prospective study using daily screening, early diagnosis and continuous monitoring *J Pain Symptom Manage* **19**, 412–26.

16 Spruyt, O. and Kausae, A. (1998). Antibiotic use for infective terminal respiratory secretions. *J Pain Symptom Manage* **15**, 263–4.

17 Macleod, A. D. (2002). Neurogenic pulmonary edema in palliative care. *J Pain and Symptom Manage* **23**, 154–6.

18 Fainsinger, R. L., Waller, A., Bercovici, M. *et al.* (2000). A multicentre international study of sedation for uncontrolled symptoms in terminally ill patients. *Pall Med* **14**, 257–65.

19 Billings, J. A. and Block, S. D. (1996). Slow euthanasia. *J Palliat Care* **12** (4), 21–30.

20 Quill, T. and Byock, I. (2000). ACP-ASIM end-of-life care consensus panel. Responding to intractable terminal suffering: the role of terminal sedation and voluntary refusal of food and fluids. *Ann Intern Med* **132**, 408–14.

21 Cherny, N. I. and Portenoy, R. K. (1994). Sedation in the management of refractory symptoms: Guidelines for evaluation and treatment. *J Palliat Care* **10** (2), 31–8.

Further reading

Baile, W. F., Buckman, R. *et al.* (2000). SPIKES-A Six-step protocol for delivering bad news: application to the patient with cancer. *The Oncologist* **5**, 302–11.

Doyle, D. and Hanks, G. (ed.) (1998). *Oxford textbook of palliative medicine* (2nd edn). Oxford: Oxford University Press.

Twycross, R., Wilcock, A., Thorp, S. (1998). *Palliative care formulary.* Radcliffe Medical Press. Therapeutic Guidelines Palliative Care Version 1, 2001. Therapeutic Guidelines Ltd, Australia.

Index

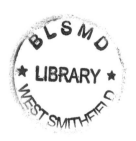